PRAISE FOR *CHANGE OF HEART*

"Sometimes in life we find ourselves cast into a trial that threatens to consume us with hopelessness, despair, and death. In these difficult seasons it can be hard to believe in a better future and a return to a life of peace, joy, and happiness. In her book, *Change of Heart*, Lori Sheldon lets us walk beside her on just such a journey as she shares the story of living through the pain, fear, and looming doubts surrounding her husband's heart transplant saga, trusting God for His provision and healing, and ultimately experiencing the breakthrough to restoration on the other side of the struggle. I highly encourage you to read this book. Whether you're currently in a difficult season of life or enjoying a time of relative peace, this book will help you see the hand of a loving God above it all working things out for your good."

—JON SANDERS, Co-Founder of EntrePastors

"If Lori's goal in *Change of Heart* was to write the book she needed to read when faced with the life or death decision of her husband's need for a heart transplant, her success will be marked by the many readers who find her book in their time of need. She avows, "When you pray, the right people show up." Just as those people showed up for Lori, Kevin, and the Sheldon family, I foresee Lori's sublime achievement when the Sheldons show up for that person, praying in a waiting room, who turns to the end table and finds *Change of Heart*."

—RANDY HANZEN, Retired Teacher

"Lori provides a raw and honest look at facing a health crisis alongside a loved one. Throughout the journey, her faith and trust in her creator shines through. An inspirational story of challenge, love and devotion to family and God."

—DR. AMANDA TULK, Chiropractor

"Lori Sheldon understands what it means to persevere when life's most difficult season hits. She shares her emotional journey as a caregiver through her husband's heart transplant. *Change of Heart* gives encouragement and guidance for those struggling with uncertainty and waiting by offering lessons Lori learned, providing scriptures of strength and the importance of leaning on others. Lori shares what it feels like to trust God with her whole heart."

—DIANE NICHOLS, Retired Teacher and Friend

"I read this book in one sitting. Lori's strong faith is what kept her strong. I may be biased, as I can picture her family when I read the words: so beautifully written, including hearing from their daughters. This book is sweet, honest and bold. Loved it!"

—KELLIE DUNCAN-NIENKERK, Friend

"Lori's book is raw and inspirational. She genuinely communicates all the ups and downs of Kevin's transplant journey. I was gripped by every page as Lori would go from her transparent struggles to self-deprecating humor. Just as it is in her life, Lori's Christian faith is woven throughout this story. I am proud to have called Lori and Kevin friends for 30 years. I believe this book will be a blessing to any reader—and a "must read" for families going through a transplant."

—BILL KINNAN, Retired Pastor

"I am honored to recommend this book to encourage you in your journey. Whether you are the caregiver of a patient, or a medical provider, you will be inspired and encouraged to make a difference in someone else's life. You may be the "light" someone needs at just the right moment, or to make it through a prolonged journey."

—M. GREGORY DESAUTEL, MD, MBA

"*Change of Heart* isn't just a chronicle of one family's medical crisis: It's a raw, honest love letter to resilience, humor, and unwavering faith. This isn't a dry medical saga; it's a whirlwind ride through emotions, from the gut-punch of Kevin's diagnosis to the rollercoaster of waiting, surgeries, and recovery. Lori's wit shines even in the darkest moments, reminding us that laughter is sometimes the best medicine—even in the sterile halls of a hospital.

This book isn't just for believers, though faith is a strong thread. It's for anyone who has ever faced a seemingly insurmountable challenge, anyone who has ever questioned God, and anyone who has clung to hope against all odds. It's a reminder that even in the darkest moments, light can find a way through, and that love, laughter, and unwavering spirit can carry us through the most brutal storms.

Get ready to laugh, cry, and hold your breath as you turn the pages of *Change of Heart*. Lori's story will stay with you long after you finish the book: a testament to the power of love, faith, and the human spirit in the face of the unpredictable."

—HEATHER KITTELSON, Founder of Fortitude, LLC

"*Change of Heart* is for anyone seeking hope in difficult times. Lori's mix of storytelling with excerpts from her daily journal paint a vivid picture of her husband Kevin's heart transplant and their family's emotional ride through the journey. The Sheldons faced so many uncertainties, but always trusted God's plan for them. Whether you're facing a heart transplant or any other hurdle in life, this book illustrates how faith can carry you through."

—LONNIE NICHOLS, Emmy Award
Winning Senior Photo/Video Specialist

"This is a beautiful account of a tumultuous transplant journey and the strength of family, faith and friends. What a great resource for anyone going through this experience! I couldn't stop reading it."

—CAROLYN STEINBORN, Friend

"In a world that seems to grow darker by the day, it's encouraging to read a book like *Change of Heart*. In our faith journey we learn that God never promised "easy." He did, however, promise he would never leave us or forsake us. This book is a testimony to just that. God is steadfast in his love for us in the valley and on the mountain top and this book is a bold reminder of that. Lori's light shines in this book, and people in the world need it more than they know."

—**JACINTA THOMPSON**, Vice President,
Retirement Plan Consulting

"This is a story about adversity, love, and faith. The events that happened show how caring for one another and trusting in God's plan can bring peace and comfort in the most challenging times. If you are walking through adversity or a challenging time, this book can inspire you to be still and know that He is God."

—**TROY BELDEN**, Chief Operating and
Technology Officer, CareTalk

"This story is remarkable. An extremely honest, relatable, and raw account of an encounter with the unthinkable, this book is a must-read for anyone passing through a family health crisis. You will not only feel seen throughout its pages but also be met with familiarity in the depths of the unknown; you will be inspired to read God's Word and trust it in your own story."

—**ABIGAIL VAN PEURSEM**, Poetice, CEO

"In this poignant narrative of Kevin and Lori's journey through a heart transplant, the book delves into the intricate emotions surrounding their journey. As her husband faces the uncertainties of the transplant, you feel Lori's commitment to her family and how faith can be both strengthened and shaken while on this emotional rollercoaster. The book captures the intricacies of the medical process, but also beautifully illustrates how faith becomes a guiding force amidst the challenges. Their story becomes a testament to the transformative power of love, resilience, and the unwavering belief that miracles can emerge even in the most uncertain moments."

—**JESSIE SCHMIDT,** Vice President, Better
Business Bureau, South Dakota

"Life's narrative often chooses us more than we choose it, and Lori Sheldon's *Change of Heart* is a poignant testament to this truth. In this compelling book, Lori shares the journey of her husband's heart transplant, weaving a story of resilience and hope. Her ability to blend depth with a sense of levity makes every page both moving and uplifting. This book is not just a story: It's an inspiration, showcasing the power of embracing life's challenges with courage. It's a must-read for anyone looking to find strength in adversity and joy in the journey of life."

—**LON STROSCHEIN,** Author of *The Trade*

"Few books tell the story from a caregiver's or loved one's perspective. As a physician, I am always focused on the patient and sometimes forget the toll that caregiver responsibilities can exact. These roles are extremely difficult, have no clear map, and often require flexibility, patience and acceptance. Lori's experience, prayers, and lessons learned remind people that they don't need to have all the answers. It's okay to feel inadequate and frustrated—even weary or resentful sometimes. It is a good reminder that the patient is not alone in the process, and open communication among the whole care team is vital for the healthy recovery of the entire family unit."

—**SHELLEY HALL,** MD, FACC, FHFSA, FAST
Chief of Transplant Cardiology and Mechanical Support/
Heart Failure at Baylor University Medical Center

CHANGE *of* HEART

CHANGE *of* HEART

Learning to Trust the Wait During
My Husband's Heart Transplant Journey

LORI SHELDON

*I dedicate this book to my mother, Adella, and my
mother-in-law, Evelyn. They provided the sweet and
salty that shaped me into the wife I am today.*

*I also dedicate this book to caregivers living the daily grind of
uncertainty. You are not alone. You have been given an opportunity
to serve a purpose laid out especially for you. I am one of you.*

TABLE OF CONTENTS

FOREWORD

This book is about my brother, Kevin Sheldon. His wife, Lori, shares the journey of him going from a healthy man to a heart transplant recipient—with little to no warning. If you find yourself in a season of uncertainty, feeling completely helpless, then you need to read this book. My sister-in-law wrote it for you.

As Kevin's brother, I was a witness to many aspects of his heart transplant journey. I am a research scientist working at one of the largest medical device companies in the world (Medtronic Inc.). I have been deeply involved in the research and development of cardiac devices for approximately 30 years, which gave me a unique perspective into my brother's situation. I knew that many heart-related problems involve "band-aids" to alleviate problems, but often do not result in cures. Likewise, I knew that the physicians were almost without exception highly dedicated and caring people, but they are not omnipotent and there is only so much they can do. Because of this I could help interpret many of the confusing aspects of Kevin's cardiac sarcoidosis, but I was still powerless to actually help.

Kevin and I come from an athletic background. Just give us a training regimen and we will follow it. Kevin tried to stay active as his heart failure progressed. Up to nearly the end, I was amazed at how briskly he would walk with such poor heart function. But there was no training plan that could defeat cardiac sarcoidosis. A new heart was needed.

From my perspective, Lori's administrative talents and diligence made it appear that she was always in control, although I am sure she was often overwhelmed. Lori's faith is present throughout the book, but this is not an overtly religious book: It is a simple and uplifting recount of her journey.

Throughout the story Lori marvels at the support she is given at key moments, but perhaps she underestimates her own part in it. When you have good healthcare, when you have spent a lifetime creating an expansive friend group, when you have a close-knit family, when you work with and listen to experienced and dedicated nurses and doctors, people will show up for you. Lori lived the journey. She was the bedrock of her family. This is her story.

— **TODD SHELDON**, Senior Distinguished
Scientist, Medtronic (Retired)

PROLOGUE

The book you have in your hands outlines how our family made it through the unthinkable: A heart transplant. When my husband was sick, I longed for encouragement and hope. I was desperate to hear and believe that everything "could" be okay. Right or wrong, I wanted advice and proof from someone who had been in my shoes: someone on this side of Heaven. Truth be told, I really didn't find it. So I decided to write it myself—for the person who is wearing those shoes now.

I often say, *I wrote the book I needed to read.*

This book is my husband's story … my story … our family's story. But most of all, it's God's story. May it serve as encouragement to you should you ever find yourself in the passenger seat and hanging on for dear life.

Chapter 1

THE DAY TIME STOOD STILL

It was a Friday morning in March of 2018. I had a coffee chat scheduled with my daughter, Bobbi, over the phone. We often pre-planned our conversations so we could both set aside the time, and I looked forward to catching up with her. My husband, Kevin, woke up that morning feeling sick. He was sweating, vomiting, and trembling. I never really worried about him having a "heart attack" but his appearance included all the tell-tale signs I'd heard of.

I know the rush-to-the-hospital drill: Get the red backpack and start throwing things together for a trip to the emergency room. Make sure to bring his meds. Don't forget the phone charger. Put protein bars in my purse for later. Bring the binder—it has all our necessary documents and prescription information in it. My gut tells me I should probably call an ambulance. I had to make a split-second decision. Do I drive or do I call 911? I really don't want the neighbors to see an ambulance at our house so I will just drive. While holding the puke bucket, Kevin tells me to just get the car started, and he will make a run for it from his recliner.

We made it to the ER. He was sick. I did everything I could to remain calm while driving, but I regretted my decision not to call an ambulance as soon as we got in the car. I pulled up to the emergency entrance, shoved the car in park, and ran inside to the registration desk. "My husband has a history of V-tach, and he is having an episode now!" I blurted out. A nurse came out of nowhere, ran to the car, and had him in a wheelchair within minutes.

Kevin's vitals did not look good. His heart was in a dangerous irregular rhythm and his blood pressure was dropping. The first attempt at shocking his heart did not work. They shocked him a second time with no time for any anesthesia. At one point, there were so many people standing around his bed, there was no room for me. I stood out in the hallway paralyzed by fear; so much so that I couldn't even pray.

My wonderful life with my husband and my girls seemed to flash before my eyes. Everything else stood still.

Chapter 2

MY WONDERFUL LIFE

Baby of the Family

I am the product of mature parents. My mother was 46 when she gave birth to me. My dad was 50. My siblings were 25 and 18 when I came into the world. My parents owned and operated a cafe in a small town at the time. A new baby was certainly not in their plan. As I grew up, I always thought it would be great to have siblings close to my age, but ultimately, I was raised more like an only child. I was a little bit spoiled and never really learned to share.

There were many benefits to having older parents. They were financially stable; their marriage was rock solid; they had plenty of time to keep an eye on me, and I received a lot of personal attention. My mother was a bit overprotective, but my dad always seemed to balance her out. My dad was a perfect "girl dad." He was quiet, but strong. He was funny, but serious when necessary. He could fix anything—or at least make a legitimate attempt. He was slow to anger, but when he got mad, we all knew he meant it.

My dad died when I was 26 years old. I had been married for only six months at the time. He died of lung cancer. Losing my dad at such a young age rocked my world. I was hit with the harsh reality of life's fragile nature. It was devastating. My mom had a hard time adjusting to my dad's death and to being alone. Watching her move through those first months and years without my dad was hard for my siblings and me. Soon after my dad passed away, my mom moved to Sioux Falls and lived near me. She became a huge part of our lives as we raised our three daughters. My mom died 23 years later at the age of ninety-four. I often wondered how different it would have been if my dad had lived longer and my mom had not lived near me. It takes a village to raise children, and I needed her. I am forever grateful for her and the strong foundation my parents provided us.

As a child I often prayed a simple prayer, "Lord, please do not take my parents until I am okay on my own."Throughout my life I knew I had older parents and feared losing them. I often wondered who I would live with if my parents died. I would cry just thinking about it. Looking back I recognize God's faithfulness to me in hearing and answering my prayer.

Opposites Attract

My husband, Kevin, is the oldest of three children. He has first-born tendencies and I am the baby of the family. That's a fun combination to build a future on. The house Kevin grew up in is less than two miles from where we have lived for over 25 years.

His parents provided him a wonderful childhood that included a stay-at-home mom and a military dad.

As a child, Kevin's free time was spent on a bicycle or playing endless games of baseball with his brother and the neighborhood kids. He ran track in high school and college. He loves to compete. He can recall times and locations of track meets as if they were yesterday. After college, he transitioned into weightlifting and spent many hours in the gym.

I met Kevin in a bar on a Monday night in a blizzard—not the ideal place for a small-town Christian girl to meet the man of her dreams, but it all worked out. When we started dating, he was a career college student with three degrees and a part time job. He was living at home with his parents where his mom made him omelets every morning. He never missed a workout and I was attracted to his incredible discipline and sense of humor.

He broke my collar bone during a playful "wrestling match" after one month of dating. My parents met him for the first time in the hospital after my shoulder surgery. It wasn't the best first impression, considering my mom was suspicious of this new boyfriend who had injured me during a wrestling match.

It only took a few years and a couple kids for my mom to warm up to my husband. From then on she called him "Kevey" and loved spoiling him with his favorite meat and potatoes meal.

A Man of Routine

Though I have never called him Kevey, my admiration for him grew with each year of our marriage. He is kind, committed, and loves routine. These qualities make him a great dad, employee, and husband.

Every time I was pregnant, Kevin wanted a boy. Every time, we got a girl! And he wouldn't trade them for the world. Our daughters are all very fond of their dad. He is big and strong with quirky humor, which makes him the fun parent.

Kevin has worked for the same company for over 35 years. His job requires numbers, relationships, and meeting deadlines. It can be stressful, but he rarely brings that home. His two-hour sessions at the gym after work every day is the perfect buffer between work and home. It also makes him a very healthy person, which I am so thankful for.

Hence, you can imagine our surprise when, in 2013, a doctor tested Kevin's heart and detected an unusual heart rhythm. We figured it must be a mistake because Kevin had no symptoms. The echocardiogram, which measures the percentage of blood leaving your heart each time it contracts, determined his ejection fraction at 65%. Since 65% is completely normal, we weren't too worried.

In October of 2014, Kevin was working in the garden and experienced an uncomfortable racing heart episode. The high heart rate continued into the next day when he went to see the doctor. The doctor at the clinic recognized the symptoms as atrial fibrillation (Afib) which describes the heart's upper chambers beating chaotically and irregularly out of sync with its lower chambers. The doctor sent him to the hospital where they performed an electrical cardioversion (they shocked him).

During the hospital stay, he underwent an angiogram procedure to determine the level of potential blockages which may require stents. No blockages were found, therefore no stents at this time. However, his ejection fraction had declined to 30%. This was cause for concern. What happened?

We were so naïve—and I'm glad we were. It almost seemed like a joke when they prescribed blood pressure and cholesterol meds to this very healthy guy. We went on with our normal life with very little thought given to this little "heart episode." The more we talked to other people, we realized Afib is pretty common and that made it seem not that scary. Our lives were busy, which sort of made us think we didn't have time for doctor appointments and hospitals right now. We did our best to put this behind us and move on.

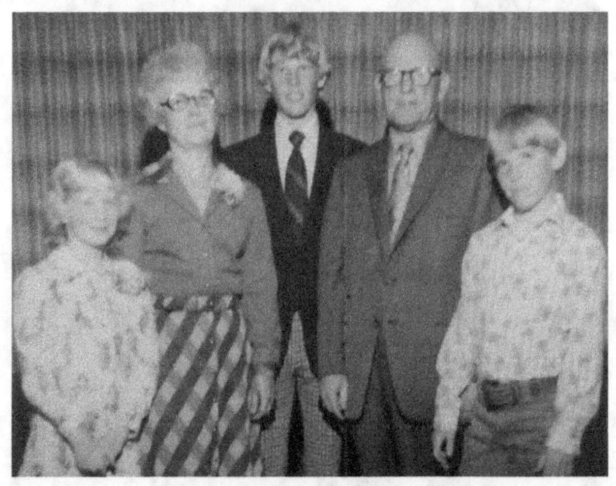

Kevin's family, 1974.

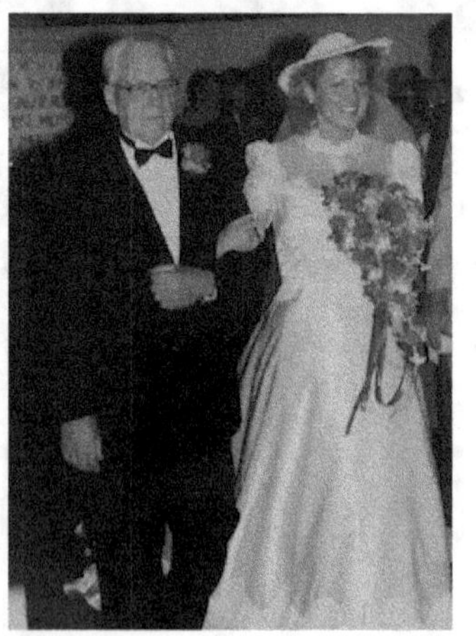

Lori's family, 1970.

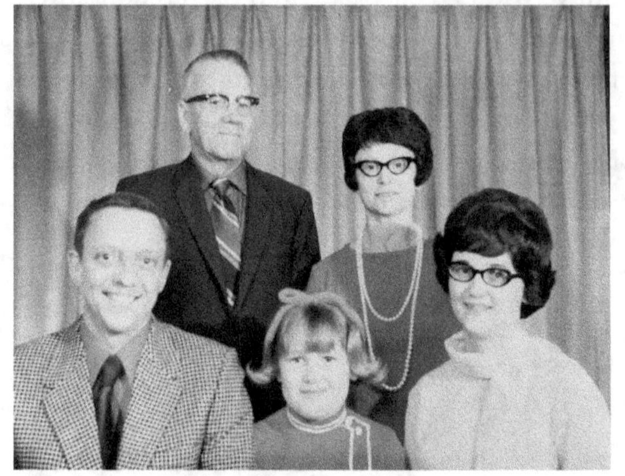

My dad and me on my wedding
day, 1987. He's so handsome!

Chapter 3

ACCEPTING THE REALITIES

Nagging Symptoms

The idea of moving on without much thought worked pretty well for me because I was not the one feeling the incidents of lightheadedness and fatigue. Kevin, on the other hand, didn't find it as easy. During an early spring fishing trip in April of 2016, he had an episode. His rapid heart rate flared up; he felt lightheaded and faint, and experienced numbness in his right hand. I probably should have been with him, but I wasn't—for two reasons. One, I was in denial that anything terrible could really be wrong with him. And two, I had vowed never to ice fish again after going once and freezing my feet off in fashion boots. Not my best decision.

Thankfully, despite his symptoms, Kevin finished the fishing trip safely but went to see his doctor when he got home. He underwent a CT scan which revealed nothing. The numbness in his hand lingered for months and became quite annoying.

A few months later, Kevin was back in the doctor's office to discuss the ongoing random episodes. The symptoms were the same: lightheadedness, feeling unwell, and rapid heart rate. An EKG was performed and reviewed by a cardiologist while we waited in the doctor's office.

Kevin and I had driven separate vehicles to this particular doctor's appointment. When the doctor advised us Kevin needed to be admitted to the hospital immediately, we had a small problem. Do we leave one vehicle here and go right to the hospital? Is it safe for Kevin to drive home and drop off his car? We discussed the problem in the parking lot and decided to both drive home so Kevin could shower. We would then proceed to the hospital. Kevin wanted answers regarding his recent episodes but being admitted to the hospital was not all that appealing. Crazy, isn't it? We thought our lives were too busy for a trip to the hospital. Thankfully, we made it home safely and I packed a small overnight bag for Kevin while he showered.

We calmly drove to the hospital and worked through the admitting process with the front office personnel. A hospital volunteer came as we completed the paperwork and walked us to Kevin's room. The medical professionals hooked Kevin up to all the necessary monitoring equipment. His nurse informed us of the tests/procedures being ordered for him.

Little did we know that this nurse would be one of many that we would see, depend on, and get to know during the journey ahead. We've come to love nurses. I'll even go so far as to say we believe nurses are doing the Lord's work. In our opinion, nurses are the best part of being stuck in a hospital. I'll be honest, though: There were times I came off as very stern, or even rude to the doctors and nurses. Kevin takes great pride in being a nice patient. He loves to get to know the nurse's own story and make a connection with them in some way. At times, Kevin's kindness could be viewed as passivity. To make certain he received the best care and that his kindness wasn't taken advantage of, I needed to play the role of the bad guy. I didn't enjoy being the "heavy," but if that's what it took for Kevin to receive the best care, I was willing to do it.

Sinking In

The first procedure that Kevin underwent was another angiogram. The test showed two blocked arteries, so the doctor inserted two stents.

During this hospital stay we were introduced to a new term. Kevin was being monitored and an irregular heart rhythm called V-tach was detected. The official name is ventricular tachycardia; it is caused by irregular electrical signals in the lower chambers of the heart. The V-tach episodes would set off an alarm at the nurse's station, and they would hurry into his room. Their reaction always got my attention and scared me. They seemed quite concerned and asked him questions like, "Kevin, are you still with us, are you okay?"

Those words finally made everything sink in. It didn't matter that Kevin was in great shape and didn't look sick. The truth was he was very ill and this was very serious. It was time to stop pretending that my husband was invincible and open my eyes to the realities of the situation.

The first reality was that in serious health situations, there are a lot of doctors, nurses, and people involved. This stressed me out at the time, but I realize now that God was just watching over us and giving us the exact people we needed, precisely when we needed them. Proof of this was Kevin's younger brother Todd, who lived four hours from us. He has spent his entire career in medical research, and one of his many specialties is the implantable cardioverter defibrillator (ICD). I usually just call the device a pacemaker, but Todd corrects me.

When I called Todd and told him they were putting a pacemaker in Kevin to help with irregular rhythm issues, Todd said, "I will be right there."

Todd and Kevin are very much alike. The way they talk and laugh, you can hardly tell them apart. They finish each other's sentences. They like the same dumb movies and history stuff. When we play family games, they cannot be on the same team because, together, they are unbeatable. Best of all, Todd has loved Kevin even longer than I have. Truly, we couldn't have asked for a better teammate to come alongside us in this situation than Todd. What a God thing.

Todd arrived within hours. His very calm demeanor was just what we needed. Heart issues can be complex and hard to comprehend but he was able to simplify the situation for us, which put some of our worries at ease. He knew the lingo and helped us understand how the pacemaker would work. Perhaps best of all, his knowledge of implantable devices meant he had influence. Needless to say, we were assured that Kevin would receive the "Cadillac" model of an ICD.

And he did. Kevin's pacemaker was put in, we received all the necessary education about it, and we learned how to send readings to the clinic as needed. He was released from the hospital with two new stents and a pacemaker. We were set! The only downside was from then on, he couldn't go through metal detectors. So making our way through airport security and concert venues would take a little longer. We decided we could live with that minor inconvenience.

Chapter 4

DIFFERENT WORRIES

Not Being There

After we returned home, life went on as normal. Kevin's heart issues seemed to be under control and managed. But there was always an underlying worry, for both me and our daughters. And we all worried about different things. This would be reality number two.

Our oldest daughter, Bobbi, had attended college at South Dakota State University, which is a short one-hour drive from our home. After college she moved back to Sioux Falls where she worked for a couple of years. Then the sad-but-happy day came when she decided to spread her wings. As a journalist, she dreamed of working in a larger news market. When an opportunity in Denver, CO, was presented to her, she jumped on it.

She sold everything she owned except for the few things that would fit in her 97 Ford Taurus. Early on a Monday morning in May 2015, about a year before Kevin received his pacemaker, she pulled out of our driveway headed for Denver. The Taurus had seen better days. It needed new brakes, and overall, it wasn't trustworthy enough for the road trip, but she made it. It was one of the proudest days of my life, yet I cried the whole day. I wanted her to pursue her dreams, but I had also become accustomed to having her nearby. We had developed routines together like long walks and Friday morning coffee chats in my kitchen. We loved shopping together and sharing clothes; I was feeling a huge void.

At the time Bobbi moved, Kevin's health issues seemed under control and managed. As time went on, I tried to keep her as informed as I could without creating unnecessary worry for her. But the distance was hard and her biggest worry was not being there should he pass away suddenly. She described it this way:

Bobbi: I've always been close with my dad. As a tomboy growing up, I preferred playing sports or going on fishing trips to piano lessons and girly things, and that meant spending lots of time outside making memories with dad. But as I got older, my mom was always the first one I wanted to tell big life updates to or have long phone calls with.

When I moved to Denver and was told about his early health episodes, I remember not being terribly concerned because he was an overall healthy guy who took care of himself. That lack of concern would be short lived.

In April 2016, the whole family made a trip out to visit for Easter and the higher elevation coupled with a declining heart made for several noticeable blips in the trip. He got light headed walking up the stairs to Red Rocks (but hey, lots of people do) and it was becoming increasingly obvious he was starting to feel overall unwell.

We still managed to have a nice trip filled with laughter, good food and mountain views.

Not long after that trip, I remember getting the call that my dad would need a pacemaker. This was accompanied by a feeling of relief that it would likely be the solution to the strange heart rhythm issues he'd been having.

This was the start of a long series of health updates I'd get throughout the next few years, almost none of which seemed good or promising.

A few months after the pacemaker had been implanted, my parents made another trip out to Denver for the 4th of July. It was a memorable trip with my dad in relatively good health. His pacemaker had him feeling better for a short time. I remember showing them favorite spots around my new neighborhood and attempting to watch fireworks from the park next to my apartment.

That would be my parents' last trip out to visit for more than three years.

Shortly after that trip, priorities shifted more urgently to when I could catch a weekend flight home or make the road trip back for a few days to visit.

Phone calls home became more frequent, and I was starting to feel scared that I could lose my dad suddenly and wouldn't be there to say goodbye. Not being there day to day to know how sick he was or what was going to happen next left me feeling helpless. "Out of sight out of mind" doesn't work when your family is close knit.

I hated knowing my daughters were worried. I felt a responsibility to keep him alive, for my daughter's sake. I couldn't let myself think about the possibility that my girls could lose their dad.

Not Qualified

For one year after the stents and pacemaker, our day-to-day life was relatively normal. We had learned to appreciate the mundane. The quiet times allowed us to enjoy a few of life's simple pleasures. We traveled to Cancun with our friends, took a family road trip to see Bobbi in Denver, planted a garden, and continued to go to work every day. I was beyond thankful for these quiet times for the obvious reasons. But the less obvious reason was this: I knew what to do. After each "normal" day, I sighed with relief that Kevin didn't need me to come through in some big way. Deep down, I worried that if I had to, I might fail.

In the summer of 2017, this worry would be put to the test.

It was a normal June Friday morning. Kevin was at his desk in the Quotations Department of Graybar Electric. He stood up to walk to his boss's office and a V-tach episode hit. He tried to wait it out, breathe, relax but it was a bad one. His boss, Chad, decided to drive him to the hospital. I got the call while on a morning walk with friends. My first thought was, "I will finish my walk and make my way to the hospital after that." It was my brain's way of calming me down by thinking, "This is no big deal."

Once I had relayed the news to my walking friends, I changed my mind and decided to get to the hospital immediately. I met Kevin at the emergency room, and the medical professionals were busy assessing his situation. Based on data from the pacemaker, he had been in an extended episode of V-tach, but the pacemaker had done its job and paced him out of it. He was stable and the heart was back to normal rhythm.

After his condition had been evaluated, he was admitted for observation. Considering the recent episode, another angiogram was performed. The stents looked good and there was no indication of further blockages. However, he had several episodes of V-tach before and after the angiogram.

Kevin handled the crazy arrhythmia episodes better than I did. They completely scared me. Each time they happened, the scary alarms would go off and the hospital staff would run into the room with the crash cart waiting outside. I would just stand there, frozen with fear, not knowing what to do, or how and when it might resolve.

Thankfully, I didn't need to know all the answers. There was someone much more qualified than I was to help, and his name was Dr. Scott Pham. He is a cardiologist and a cardiac electrophysiologist, specializing in the electrical activity of the heart. Dr. Pham briefly discussed with us possible treatments for arrhythmia including something called an "ablation." We noted what he said, spent three more days at the hospital, and then Kevin was released to go home.

That's when I realized, I didn't want to take him home! I had zero medical experience, barely knew what ablation meant, and didn't know the first thing to do if another V-tach episode were to occur. I had always felt completely capable of balancing a few balls and wearing a few different hats, per se, but this? No way. I was completely overwhelmed: completely unqualified for this endeavor. But the reality was, I had to figure it out. I was his wife.

So I got the keys out of my purse, retrieved the vehicle, and parked in front of the sliding hospital doors. The nurse wheeled him out and helped him into the car. For the time being, he'd be all mine. For better or for worse, in sickness or in health.

The next morning, my devotions read, "*The problem with an easy life is, it masks the need for God.*"

There He was again, reminding me I was not alone on this journey. We were not alone.

Chapter 5

NOT MAKING SENSE

Mark Steinborn

Kevin studied and ran track at South Dakota State University from 1976 to 1979. He became lifelong friends with many people during that season in life. One was Mark Steinborn.

I've said it often, "Everyone needs a Mark Steinborn in their life." Mark was one of a kind, had a wild sense of humor and a goofy personality, and was an absolute rock star at his life's work, which was a certified registered nurse anesthetist (CRNA). Mark and Kevin fished together, played on the same softball team, and enjoyed living just two blocks apart from each other. I didn't realize it at the time, but even this detail—being neighbors—was ordained. Just like Todd, Mark was an answer to my prayers.

It was a Friday night in July 2017 and Jazz Fest in Sioux Falls was going on. We were home because Kevin wasn't feeling well, and I was a bit annoyed because everyone I knew was enjoying the live music event. We were getting to the point where it was hard to make plans because we never knew how Kevin would feel.

I was uneasy with Kevin's symptoms and needed a little reinforcement, so I decided to call Mark. I was surprised he was home as I thought he would surely be at Jazz Fest with everyone else. Mark came immediately with a stethoscope and performed a basic assessment. Within 10 minutes, the three of us were in the car on the way to the ER. I drove and Mark rode in the back seat. Kevin rode shotgun. We were all quiet the entire drive to the hospital.

Once again Kevin was shocked back to normal rhythm. Mark hung around the hospital with me for several hours. It was comforting to have a medical person by my side when the crazy was happening. At one point we had to be out of the room, so Mark and I were hanging out in the hallway and a person walked by and said something to us. We both nodded and smiled. Mark turned to me and said, "What did he say?" I had no idea. We both laughed about our old age hearing loss and how we just shook our heads "yes" and agreed.

Kevin remained in the hospital for the weekend. Dr. Pham revisited the conversation with us regarding an ablation procedure. He reminded us that cardiac ablation is done using a catheter, creating tiny scars in the heart to block irregular electrical signals in an effort to correct arrhythmias. The success rate he described wasn't great, but we were in need of possible solutions.

The next morning during my morning devotions, I sensed the Lord telling me, *"You think this is the end, but it is really just the beginning of something new."*

First Ablation: August 2017

A month later at our follow up visit with Dr. Pham, we decided to proceed with the ablation procedure. The first one was done in August. The procedure lasted about five hours. I had an army of support around me in the waiting room for the day. Todd and his wife, Missy, came from Minneapolis. Our youngest two daughters, Brooke and Regan, were also there. And Bobbi was praying from Denver. We made the best of a long day of waiting.

Dr. Pham met with us in a consultation room after the procedure, still wearing his full scrub gear and reported to me his frustration. He was unable to induce the V-tach during the procedure which made his efforts in mapping the correct location very difficult. During this conversation Dr. Pham mentioned the term "heart failure" to us. Kevin's brother, Todd, assured me it was a broad term describing many heart-related issues but it was a real punch in the gut for us to hear.

Kevin went home with little success. He continued to have an overall feeling of fatigue, in and out of V-tach, unable to work out at the gym—which is his lifeblood—and continued to go to work as he could, which was sporadically. Thankfully, his boss and his fellow employees were very supportive and picked up the slack—a reminder that being loyal and having good relationships at work is very important.

During this time, I felt helpless. So I did the only thing I knew in my heart to do: pray big and pray boldly.

"God, please. I don't care how, but somehow heal Kevin's 'trick' heart. I can't comprehend how you'll do this, but I promise to give you all the credit."

A deep peace came over me after I prayed, gave God complete control, and asked Him to completely heal Kevin's heart. Shortly thereafter, I stumbled upon Ezekiel 36:26, which read, *"And I will give you a new heart and put a new spirit within you."* The words spoke to my soul, and again I felt a peace and a confidence that came from somewhere bigger than me. I believed God had a path leading us to healing. I just needed to trust. I told myself, *"This story has already been written, I just need to live it."*

Now I needed Kevin to believe the promise. I went to the computer and printed several copies of the verse and put them in pretty picture frames. I placed them all over the house. I strategically placed it on his bathroom counter, on his nightstand, in the kitchen, and in our family room. I made it the screensaver on my IPAD for me to see each time I went to Dr. Google for answers. It would remind me of the promise from the Great Physician.

Believing the Doctor, Believing the Promise

For the next couple weeks, we had follow-up visits with Dr. Pham. During one of these, he mentioned two words I never thought I'd hear in my life: heart transplant. They sounded ridiculous to me. For a brief time, I reverted back to my old self and avoided reality. I told myself that there is no way we are heading in that extreme direction. I had never heard or known of anyone who had a heart transplant; there must be some mistake.

Yet I knew Dr. Pham was an excellent doctor. He is well respected and even though we experienced little success under his care, we trusted him and listened to what he advised us to do. I asked his nurse during an appointment, "Do you guys have any success with your work? Because we are not seeing it." She smiled and said, "Oh, yes! We see a lot of success."

When we returned home from the appointment, I opened my IPAD and the first thing I saw was the verse from before,

Ezekiel 36:26, *"And I will give you a new heart and put a new spirit within you."* There it was again, the promise from God. I thought to myself, *"It's simple. I have the promise. I just need to believe it."*

I turned to Kevin on the other end of the couch and said, *"You know what? You are going to get a new heart from a wonderful donor! We will meet the family one day and show them what good care you are taking of their beloved heart."* I still thought the whole idea was ridiculous but saying it out loud gave me a little peace. I needed to find hope somehow, somewhere.

Kevin replied, *"Whatever."*

That weekend we rented a movie "The Case for Christ" and watched it with our youngest daughter, Regan. The woman in the movie had chosen Ezekiel 36:26 to pray over her husband. There it was again! We all looked at each other. Could it be a coincidence?

Second Opinion

In the fall of 2017, I started a new part-time job at Garfield Elementary. Brooke taught second grade at this school, so I had an "in." I was excited to get immersed in her environment and find a spot where I could contribute.

After one day at my new job, Kevin was back in the hospital with multiple V-tach episodes. On a positive note, my new job at the school was a five-minute drive to the hospital. Once again, I met Kevin in the emergency room. During this hospital stay, Dr. Pham made a recommendation for Kevin to see one of his colleagues at the University of Minnesota, Dr. Roukoz. Dr. Pham had gone through medical school with him and was willing to make the phone call for us. We were grateful for the recommendation considering we had not given any thought to looking for another opinion at this point. We appreciated Dr. Pham admitting his own limitations and putting Kevin's needs first.

The next morning, we were making plans to head to Minneapolis. Kevin was not stable enough to travel with us, so he was airlifted there. The girls and I discussed my travel plans. Regan was attending college at SDSU at the time and looking forward to a fun trip to Denver to see Bobbi and attend a concert at Red Rocks. But she forfeited her trip so she could come with me to Minneapolis. I was grateful; her sarcastic wit, knack for relating to people, and ability to stay strong were just what I needed. Regan shared later that my calm was just what she needed.

Regan: In the early stages of my dad's illness I came home from college a lot. I wasn't overly concerned about the severity of his heart issues but in general, I'm a homebody and liked being home. I enjoyed spending time with my dad. We watched the same movies, and his weird humor aligns with mine. My sisters may disagree, but I think I'm special to my Dad.

Our family had no experience with heart-related issues so the medical terms being thrown around were all foreign to us. I followed my mom's lead, and she didn't seem overly concerned so I remained calm as well. Ignorance can be bliss at times.

My girls came through for me too many times to count. Minneapolis is a four-hour drive from our house and the thought of navigating the city by myself was more than I could take. While traveling there, Regan encouraged me to contact Gay Lynn, a friend who lived near the Cities. She was familiar with the area and agreed to meet us in a suburb and let us follow her to the University of Minnesota campus. She was the best escort, and safely got us to the front door of the hospital—valet parking and all. When you pray, people really do show up.

Todd and his son Mark were with Kevin when Regan and I found our way to his room. Mark was attending the University of Minnesota and living on campus at the time. Kevin's nurse was called Joseph, and they had already become fast friends. Kevin had met with Dr. Roukoz and an ablation procedure had been scheduled for the next morning.

Minneapolis turned out to be a complete godsend. Dr. Pham's best connections were at the University of Minnesota and the friends and family we needed weren't far away. Thank you, Lord.

Second Ablation, September 2017, University of Minnesota

Regan and I stayed at Todd and Missy's house and the next day made our way to the hospital bright and early for a day of waiting. The procedure lasted eight hours. It was a brutally long day. We spent the day watching other waiting families, with all of us constantly anticipating when our turn would come to be recruited into the consultation room. Todd, Mark, and Regan were with me the entire day.

However, when we finally were called in to talk to Dr. Roukoz and his nurse, it was just Mark and me. Todd had left briefly to attend his daughter's soccer game and Regan had slipped out to grab a coffee with her friend, Whitney. With concern on his face and kindness in his voice, Dr. Roukoz told us that Kevin's heart failure was much worse than originally thought.

He explained that Kevin's heart was pumping poorly, that the blood's dark red color was not ideal, and that they weren't able to induce Kevin's irregular heart rhythm during the procedure, making the ablation only somewhat successful at best. Dr. Roukoz was able to get some good mapping completed during the procedure, which was an accomplishment. I didn't know what that meant but it seemed to be important to the doctor.

Dr. Roukoz ended by saying, "The good news is that your husband is in excellent physical shape which may be the reason he has been able to tolerate a poor functioning heart for some time."

Once again, God gave me the right person by my side. My nephew, Mark, used his sharp mind and recalled the conversation with the doctor word for word. He later relayed it to Todd and Regan. It hit me even harder hearing it a second time in Mark's words. Basically, the news was not good.

Regan and I were allowed to visit Kevin briefly after the procedure, but he was groggy and tired. We left the hospital and spent the night at Todd and Missy's house. It was a bad night. The news from the doctor was devastating for us and Kevin was going to hear the update in the morning. I was convinced my husband was going to die. My dad died when I was 26 years old and there was a good chance that I'd have to watch my daughters lose their dad too. This wasn't fair.

Regan and I went to bed in our separate rooms. Neither of us could sleep. Eventually I made my way upstairs to lie with her and we tried to make sense of what had happened that day. We decided to not tell her sisters until we could process the news a little better ourselves. We cried. I had no desire to try and be the strong one for my daughter. I was broken and scared.

Early the next morning, we traveled back to the hospital, dreading the day ahead. Kevin wanted to know the outcome. Dr. Roukoz performed his rounds and, with a team of white coats standing around him, he laid out for my husband a bleak analysis. "Kevin, some people are born with a heart that lasts 80 years; yours will not last that long."

I couldn't even look at Kevin. We tried to ask some questions but none of them made any sense. The medical team left the room, and not one of us uttered a word. Eventually Kevin broke the silence. "Who is going to take care of my family? What will you and Regan do for insurance?" No one answered. After several minutes, Kevin whispered through tears, "I wish I could have more time with you."

Chapter 6

CARDIAC SARCOIDOSIS

Dr. Roukoz referred our case to the Heart Failure Team at the University of Minnesota. Several well-meaning professionals stopped by his room to give us brochures and high-level information on an LVAD pumping device. It was too soon. We were not in a mindset to hear or process any of this. A lovely nurse shared success stories she had experienced with other patients receiving the LVAD device. Her kindness and expertise took some of the edge off our raw emotions.

We now had to wait and see if the ablation had produced any success. Kevin was discharged the next day and we returned home to Sioux Falls. His next follow-up appointment with Dr. Pham was two weeks out. Kevin was not able to return to work. He continued to experience recurrent V-tach episodes.

Several days later, he came out of the shower one morning and immediately sat down on the steps, feeling lightheaded. Soon after he sat down, I heard an unusual moan/yell. It was a very animalistic sounding cry. Like nothing I had ever heard before. When I came around the corner from the kitchen, he was lying back on the steps and said, "I think I got shocked by my pacemaker!" This had never happened, and I didn't know what to do. Less than a minute later, he was shocked again. He made his way over to the couch to lay down and I called the nurse.

We saw Dr. Pham later that day in the clinic and determined another ablation would be necessary. It was scheduled for October 10th in Minneapolis. My birthday is October 9th. Happy birthday to me.

We traveled to Minneapolis on my birthday and Kevin was feeling awful. He was weak and any amount of activity caused irregular rhythms. While I drove, he laid the seat back and endured the four-hour drive. We stayed with Todd and Missy again while anticipating another long day and procedure ahead. Missy gave Kevin a prayer shawl. It was made with love and prayed over by her knitting group. The shawl would remain with Kevin for the next two years.

The next day, Kevin and Dr. Roukoz spent another eight-hour day together. Dr. Roukoz was more hopeful this time. He believed this time we might see better results. Time would tell.

The tricky thing about a successful ablation is the ability to induce the V-tach to give the physician a path to follow. One way to do that is to bring the patient in and out of sedation. Kevin recalls waking up during the procedure and complaining, "My back hurts." Dr. Roukoz replied, "So does mine." We still smile about that.

The next morning Dr. Roukoz stopped by Kevin's hospital room and pulled up a chair beside the bed. He said to Kevin, "On my way home last night, I was thinking about you. What could possibly be causing this healthy guy to be experiencing these symptoms? Why does this 58-year old man appear to have a very low functioning heart? Should we be testing him for cardiac sarcoidosis?" He continued, "I am part of the sarcoid team here at the U of M and I would like to run some tests." Dr. Roukoz ordered an MRI to get a preliminary look. Further testing would follow if needed. We did not know it at the time, but this was the beginning of preparing Kevin for a new heart. We returned home to Sioux Falls and Kevin recovered nicely. He went back to work two weeks later.

Once again, my morning devotions spoke to me. *When you imagine the future (worry) don't imagine what you can do—but what God will do.*

In December we received confirmation of the diagnosis: cardiac sarcoidosis. A heart biopsy and pet scan confirmed the results. Sarcoidosis is an inflammatory disease in which the immune system overreacts and causes clusters of inflamed tissue to cluster up in various parts of the body. Kevin's heart would experience flares of the sarcoid and leave behind scar tissue, which caused the irregular rhythm. Along with that, the heart did not contract like normal heart tissue, therefore his heart pumping function worsened.

The beginning treatment was high dose prednisone to attempt to calm down the sarcoid flare by reducing inflammation. By this time, I had stopped counting the number of medications Kevin had been on because there had been so many. He had been prescribed any and everything in an attempt to control the erratic heart rhythm. At one point he was on three beta-blockers. Each of them is not recommended for long term use. After a month on prednisone, he developed a blood clot in the leg and was prescribed blood thinners. By Christmas Kevin was retaining a lot of fluid and did not feel well. He was then prescribed Lasix. Because of the extra fluid, he was short of breath and his entire body was puffy. Very quickly he developed the infamous "moon face" which is common with prednisone. He no longer looked healthy.

The girls were all home for Christmas, and we made the best of a very low key time. Our family tradition is to spend the holidays with Kevin's siblings and their families. His sister, Sheila, an amazing hostess, puts on a tremendous spread for every holiday. Kevin did his best to endure the family time but on Christmas Day we opted to stay home while the girls went on ahead to the family gathering.

I'll be honest. At times I resented being stuck at home because Kevin wasn't feeling good, and this was one of those times. I kept my feelings to myself but it was hard being the healthy one and missing out. I didn't want to go to Christmas without Kevin, but I also didn't want to stay home. My feelings were all over the place.

A New Year

In January, Kevin was retaining fluid which made his breathing difficult. He had been sleeping in the recliner to be able to get any kind of rest. His face was puffy from the fluid overload, and he was wearing compression socks to help the leg swelling. It was decided that he needed to return to Minneapolis for two days of tests. Brooke was still on Christmas break and she offered to be our driver.

Brooke: I am the daughter that stayed living close to home. I love living in Sioux Falls and accept the responsibility that comes with it. I was able to be at the hospital at a moment's notice and attend a few doctor appointments with my dad. I'm grateful I could be their chauffeur when needed. My mom tends to process her emotions internally and hold her fear tightly inside which can make it difficult for me to know what to do. I was not afraid for my dad. I had a peace that it would somehow work out. Maybe I was naive, but I like to think it was the Holy Spirit.

After two days of testing, we finished up at a clinic appointment with Dr. Rebecca Cogswell. When you pray, God brings you to the right people. Dr. Cogswell is a Cardiologist, serves on the University of Minnesota Sarcoid team, is a heart failure specialist and specifically guides patients through the process of organ transplantation. We liked her immediately. She spoke with such confidence, and I loved her direct approach. She examined Kevin, reviewed his test results and put a specific plan together to get him feeling better. She slid boldly into the driver's seat to determine Kevin's course of treatment, and she made us feel hopeful!

Brooke, Kevin, and I walked out of that clinic with a skip in our step. Dr. Cogswell had prescribed a medication cocktail to "put out the fire of this sarcoid". She gave us some peace of mind by saying, "We may be able to control the sarcoid and get you feeling better, but if the time comes where a transplant is needed, I will be the one to make that call."

We went home and Kevin experienced some success with the new meds. He went back to work and the next few months were as normal and quiet as they'd been in a long time: the quiet before the storm ...

"The Friday" in March 2018

I woke up before Kevin and went into the kitchen to start the coffee. I checked my phone to make sure the volume was on;

I didn't want to miss Bobbi's call. I was looking forward to hearing her voice and catching up on the happenings of the week. But this phone call and morning didn't go as planned.

"Lori!" Kevin called my name. I went downstairs and found him in the recliner sweating, vomiting, and trembling—tell-tale signs of a heart attack.

I got the backpack and filled it with meds, the phone charger, protein bars, and "The Binder" with all our necessary documents and prescription information in it.

Ignoring my gut instinct to call an ambulance, I got in the car and backed it out of the garage. Then I ran back inside to get Kevin. He was in the recliner holding the puke bucket. On the count of three I pulled him up from the recliner and followed him up the short flight of stairs. We made it out the back door and into the car.

I did everything I could to remain calm while driving, but Kevin was vomiting and sweating profusely. I regretted my decision to not call an ambulance. I pulled up to the emergency entrance, shoved the car in park, and ran inside to the registration desk. "My husband has a history of V-tach, and he is having an episode now!" I blurted out. A nurse came out of nowhere, ran to the car, and had him in a wheelchair whizzing past me within minutes.

Kevin's vitals did not look good. He was in V-tach, and his blood pressure was dropping. The first attempt at shocking his heart did not work. They shocked him a second time. I watched from the hallway outside his room. I remained calm but knew things were not looking good. I had never seen a blood pressure this low.

Everything was surreal—even the handsome Emergency Room doctor. His good looks frightened me a bit; it was too much like the scene from one of the hospital shows. Would

"Dr. McDreamy" be coming with bad news about my husband and comfort me by putting his arm around me? I thought, "Oh no! Is this the end?"

Thankfully, no, it was not the end. Eventually they were able to manipulate Kevin's pacemaker and the device paced him back into normal rhythm. He wasn't completely out of the woods yet, but his condition was starting to look a little better.

My cell phone rang. It was Bobbi. "Hi Mom! Happy Friday!" I had to confess that—once again—I was at the hospital. I hated being a constant downer for my girls. There was no good way to spin this. He was sick again. I gave her a quick overview but had to hang up to tend to the registration paperwork.

While hanging up, I saw a person out of the corner of my eye: Pastor Jeff Heron, the associate pastor from Linwood Wesleyan Church where we'd attended for 18 years. Pastor Jeff was a dynamic "people" person with a calm demeanor who I trusted and enjoyed. Again, God's hand was at work, sending me the right person at the right time in the right place.

I updated Pastor Jeff on the situation, and he reacted in his usual reassuring way. We chatted briefly and he told me that if I needed anything, he would be there to help. It was so good to see him.

I called Regan and Brooke and they both came to the hospital. Kevin had been moved to another floor where they continued interventions to stabilize him. Dr. Pham was called in and he determined that Kevin needed to be transferred to the U of M again. Pastor Jeff made his way to Kevin's room and greeted the girls by their first names. He always remembered names! Kevin looked over at us in the corner chatting with Pastor Jeff and felt so grateful this man of God was there to care for me and his girls.

Pastor Jeff asked if he could pray with us. The girls and I stood in a huddle while Pastor Jeff covered us in prayer asking our Heavenly Father to meet all our needs and to restore Kevin to perfect health. We felt very raw and yet so loved.

Once again, Kevin traveled to Minneapolis on a Sanford Health jet. The girls and I went home to decide who would go to Minneapolis and who would stay back.

Chapter 7

DENIAL

Ablation #4

Dr. Cogswell and Dr. Roukoz determined another ablation procedure was the best course of action at this time. Once again, the procedure lasted eight hours and Dr. Roukoz gave us a somewhat positive report. I had learned to sturdy myself for the consultation meetings with the doctors. They never seemed to bear good news. Fortunately, this time Dr. Roukoz had been able to stimulate the V-tach and was able to successfully perform the ablation.

While I was in the waiting room that day, I had the opportunity to visit a 35-year-old man who had had a heart transplant three weeks earlier. Many people in the waiting room were talking to him; he was getting attention like a local hero. In my conversation with him, he told me of the requirement to live near the hospital for 30 days after the surgery for the necessary follow up and lab appointments: 30 days!! I thought that was ridiculous. Who could live away from home for a month? How would we ever do that? I was in denial. I just couldn't accept that an actual heart transplant would be in Kevin's future. I really wanted one of these procedures to do the trick so we could avoid all the drama of a heart transplant.

The next day I told Kevin about my conversation with the transplant guy. I said, "We are never going to do that. The guy didn't look great and let's just be firm with the doctors and say we are not going to do that!" I was clearly still in denial of the seriousness of the situation.

While I was wrestling with the reality of our situation, Dr. Cogswell was busy coordinating the necessary steps for evaluation of a heart transplant. She instructed the Advanced Therapies Team to begin the preliminary work up. Since Kevin was already in the hospital, they decided they might as well get the long list of necessary tests and evaluations done. It took a couple days and a tremendous amount of coordination from several specialties within the hospital, but the checklist was completed:

- CT Scan—head and chest
- Ultrasound—carotid arteries
- Artery and lower extremities scan
- Meeting with a dietician
- Meeting with LVAD coordinator to demonstrate the device
- Neurological psych test
- Meeting with a social worker
- Palliative Care Team meeting
- Examination by psychologist

For many of the meetings, I had to be there. The one with the Palliative Care Team was especially hard. It was a lot of discussion about end-of-life wishes. It forced us to have difficult conversations and I didn't like it. I sat with my arms crossed for most of it while the very kind lady prodded us for answers. Kevin cooperated nicely and reprimanded me after the meeting, saying, "You can't act like that or I'm going to get kicked out of this program because of you!"

I guess I was still in denial that this heart transplant thing was really going to happen. Who could blame me?

After 12 days in the hospital, Kevin was feeling pretty good, so they let us go home. We were welcomed into our kitchen by the aroma of soup in the crock pot. My niece, Lisa, had been watching our dogs while we were away and graciously brought them home along with the soup. I called Lisa many times with my need for an emergency dog-watching service and she was always right on it. Lisa and her family lived seven blocks from us and she never waited to be asked what she could do; she just did it.

She was wonderful. And being home was wonderful.

I read in my devotion the next morning, "God knows the future and I know God." I know now that this was not a coincidence; His words never are. God knew I was in denial and wanted to tell me everything would be okay.

Chapter 8

TIME IS TICKING

A week later we met with Dr. Pham for a clinic appointment. Dr. Pham reviewed the readings from the pacemaker and determined that Kevin had had some incidents with V-tach since the last ablation. They were minor and not always noticeable to Kevin; however, he was experiencing heaviness and bloating in his chest and abdomen. Dr. Pham ordered an echocardiogram and determined his new ejection fraction (the ability of the heart to pump blood) was now at 20%.

Dr. Pham prescribed another beta blocker to his already extensive medication regimen and did not recommend any further ablation procedures. He wanted to see Kevin every two weeks. Because of the water retention and uncomfortable bloating, the doctors also determined it was time to taper down the prednisone. Like it does with any sickness, time seemed to go so slowly: doctor appointments, medication changes, extended periods of rest, waiting for test results, et cetera. Dr. Pham described Kevin's heart failure as fast-moving, and I just remember thinking, "Really?" Perspective is an interesting thing.

Withdrawal

Within a week or so, Kevin was feeling very sick again with flu-like symptoms. Tapering off the prednisone was likely the culprit. The withdrawal reaction manifested as extreme chills, fever, sweating, loss of appetite, and lightheadedness. As caregiver, I had to decide what to do or who to call about this. I contacted both U of M and Sanford Health Teams and they recommended he see his primary physician for lab work. Infection was suspected and his primary doctor would be the best one to determine this. What the heck? He hadn't been to his primary in over two years, and he would have no idea of Kevin's current status.

This was extremely frustrating for me (and Kevin). I did as told and called to make an appointment as quickly as possible. However, his primary doctor was on vacation so the best we could do was see one of his partners that afternoon. We showed up, binder in hand.

The "new" doctor ordered lab work, which showed no infection. He expressed concern over the "medication cocktail" that he was on, which made us chuckle. We felt like saying, "Well, that makes three of us!" We left knowing Kevin's blood pressure was slightly low (which made sense) and no clear or helpful answers. Kevin returned home feeling as ill as he had before we left. By this time, both of our stomachs were uneasy.

Here We Go Again

Two days later we were preparing for Easter weekend. Our daughter Bobbi was driving home from Denver and her boyfriend Sam was with her. Sam is a South Dakota native too, so making the 10-hour drive was "coming home" for him as well. They pulled into the driveway, and I immediately greeted them with the news that Kevin was sick and we should probably take him to the ER. Welcome home.

We packed up the red backpack again and headed off to the hospital with the binder. Once Kevin was evaluated by the ER team; Dr. Pham's team was alerted. Kevin's markers looked much worse than just two days prior when they performed labs at the Family Practice Clinic. I knew what that meant: Minneapolis, here we come. I tried to convince Dr. Pham's nurse practitioner, Michelle, that since it was Easter weekend, we really wanted to stay in Sioux Falls. She sat next to Kevin's bed and kindly but firmly told us, "Kevin, if you take a turn for the worse, we are not equipped to handle it here. You need to be in Minneapolis." She had tears in her eyes. She had come to know Kevin and it was clear she cared about him. She was also nine months pregnant and ready to deliver any day so hormones may also have been a factor.

Once again Kevin was airlifted to U of M. It was Good Friday. Todd met Kevin at the hospital when he arrived. Brooke and I made the trip to Minneapolis again. Regan, Bobbi, and Sam stayed in Sioux Falls. We were always making hard decisions about who should go and who should stay. In the end, Bobbi and Sam saw Kevin for approximately two hours that Easter weekend: not exactly what we had planned.

During this stay in the hospital at the U of M we had a meeting with Kevin's Transplant Coordinator. It was nice to finally meet her after speaking with her on the phone many times. She explained the evaluation process for a transplant. Those decisions were made by a committee that met every Friday to review patient profiles. Kevin's case would be reviewed and if all went well, he would be listed for transplant. It still seemed so outrageous. I tried to view this update as good news but I still couldn't grasp the reality of it all. The coordinator was a true professional in her role and she sensed our mixed emotions. She arranged for us to meet an actual transplant patient. Her name was Traci.

Traci had had her transplant four years earlier after waiting in the hospital for nine months. She looked amazing. She was now able to live a normal life which included traveling, exercising, and planning her daughter's wedding. Wow! It was exactly what we needed to see. We heard from doctors, nurses, and other medical professionals all day long about the process but to see an actual survivor meant everything to us. Traci gave me her number and asked me to reach out to her at any time with anything we may need. I was starting to understand that we were on the road to a transplant.

Kevin remained in the hospital a bit longer for further testing. Brooke needed to get back to work and I had matters to handle on the home front. Brooke and I traveled home without Kevin. Brooke was nursing a broken heart from a recent break-up and Regan needed her wisdom teeth out. Bobbi was 10 hours away and my husband was in the hospital. I was feeling overwhelmed and tired. I needed a break from it all.

The very next day Kevin called, "Hey! Good news! I'm being released today!" My reaction was not positive. Good grief, we just left yesterday! "Why are you being released so soon?" I asked. He explained that he had finished his necessary tests and was anxious to get home. "Come and get me," he said. I told him I would see what I could do and hung up.

Regan volunteered. She made the trip to Minneapolis and brought him home.

All the required tests for transplant evaluation were complete. Now we had to wait on a decision from the committee. In my devotional, I read what it meant to surrender: It means signing the bottom of the page, and then letting the Lord fill in the blanks. Time was ticking, but I wasn't quite sure I was ready to pick up the pen.

Chapter 9

HURRY UP AND WAIT

Journal Entry: Things I Miss From My Old Life (April 3, 2018)
- *I miss walking across a parking lot with Kevin without the fear he is going to collapse*
- *I miss making travel plans with the Nichols—half the fun is making the plans*
- *I miss being able to make plans for anything!*
- *I miss seeing Kevin come home from the gym drenched in sweat*

By this point, I was struggling. I was tired of watching the rest of the world go on with their lives while we were living our lives from one doctor appointment to another. Why does Kevin have to be sick? He does not deserve this. These thoughts were only mine. Kevin was consistently brave and never questioned the unfairness of the situation. He was not afraid of receiving another man's heart. He only regretted what this was doing to his family.

On April 6, 2018, we received the news that Kevin had been listed for transplant! We were advised to answer every phone call, pack a bag, and be ready to travel to Minneapolis at a moment's notice. The girls and I created a Facebook page to keep friends and family informed. I'll admit, this was very hard on me; I hated it. It was physically painful for me to put this out to the world. It made it seem so real. I would have preferred to process my emotions quietly in a dark room by myself, and my girls are similar to me in that regard. None of us knew how to ask or receive outside help very well. This is not a good quality, and we blame it on our Dutch heritage. All that said, we knew other people cared and were praying for Kevin, too. A Facebook page was our way of letting them know how he was doing.

I must have been worn out because I came down with influenza. I was so sick. Body aches, bad cough and fever. I felt like crap, and I tried to keep my distance from Kevin so I wouldn't make him sick. I laid low for three days and then I began to reemerge back to normal life.

Kevin and I lived our lives knowing that each day that passed brought us one day closer to a new heart. We chose to trust God's perfect timing in all of this. I actually felt relief in letting go and trusting God to care for the "when." I felt a nudge during my morning devotions to anoint Kevin with oil for healing. He would probably think I was crazy. I noted in my journal, *"I wonder if I'm going to follow through with this nudge."* I also wrote this prayer, *"Use our circumstances, Lord, to be a light to someone else."*

Anointing Kevin

My nephew Cody and his wife, Kelly were full time missionaries on a college campus. They were in town and stopped by for a visit. It was a beautiful spring evening, and we were outside on the back deck. The grass was turning green, and the dark days of winter were behind us. Regan was home and we enjoyed great conversation with each of us sharing our faith journeys.

While they were there, James 5:14 kept coming to mind. *Is anyone among you sick? Let him call for the elders of the church, and let them pray over him, anointing him with oil in the name of the Lord.*

I had no idea if Kevin would be okay with this, but I finally asked Cody to anoint Kevin with oil and pray over him. Cody quickly responded that he would be happy to, so I ran in the house and grabbed the first essential oil bottle I could find. We all gathered around Kevin with our hands on his shoulders while Cody prayed. It was the perfect preparation for what was to come.

The very next Friday, Kevin was at work and started to feel ill. Once again, a co-worker, Randy, drove him to the emergency room, and I met them there. (Randy eventually told me it was the scariest ride of his life.) The Sanford Heart Team immediately began communicating with the University of Minnesota, and it was decided that Kevin needed to go to Minneapolis again. But this time, he would have to stay there . . . and wait . . . for a new heart.

I asked the flight team at the hospital if I could quickly run home, get the bags I was supposed to already have packed, and meet them at the airport. They said yes, they'd give me 30 minutes. They quickly delivered instructions for me to find the Sanford Health hangar at the airport and where to meet them.

I tried to memorize the instructions and ran to my car. I called my friend, Karen, and asked her to meet me at my house. I needed a clear-thinking mind to help me get this done quickly. Karen was already in my driveway when I got home, and we ran through the house throwing things in his suitcase. She drove me to the airport as I tried to recall the directions they'd given me.

It was raining and we arrived just before the ambulance did. I made my way out to the tarmac as they loaded Kevin onto the plane. I told Karen to take pictures for us to remember. I climbed onto the plane to give them his suitcase. I kissed Kevin goodbye and that was it. You would think I would have been a blubbering mess, but I was so relieved. So very relieved. He was being airlifted for hopefully the last time. And I was beyond ready for this chapter to end and the next one to begin.

A Quiet House

I came home to a quiet house. I sat in the quiet for a long time. What had just happened? The real wait was just beginning. I made the decision to stay home for the time being, and I have no idea how I came to that decision. For the first few days it was a relief to no longer have a sick person in my home. I removed all evidence of his medication, blood pressure cuff, stethoscope, etc. I needed our home to feel normal and cleansed of the sickness.

Kevin and I talked every day. His days were long, and he tried to be positive. He developed a walking routine on the hospital floor which gave him the opportunity to visit other heart patients.

My niece, Deb, came by my house one evening with a gift for me. During a season in her life, she had also taken on the role of caregiver when her husband was ill. He eventually lost his battle.

We sat on my deck for hours and shared our experiences with one another. It was nice to talk to someone who knew and had experienced the many emotions of a caregiver. When I told her I removed all evidence of sickness from my house she knew exactly what I meant. It was a relief to share my weird thoughts and not have to apologize for any of it.

Kevin quickly found his favorite nurses. Initially he was in a shared room with another heart patient, but the nurses all knew he wanted to move to a private room as soon as possible. Late one evening his nurse rushed into the room and told him to pack up quickly! She had a room for him. She also arranged for his own mini fridge! Kevin asked her if this was okay to be moving rooms? It was 10pm. Should we be doing this? She commented, "Around here, possession is 9/10 of the law." The private room improved his spirits tremendously. The same favorite nurse brought him broasted chicken from home. Her husband was famous for making it and she wanted Kevin to sample it.

The mini fridge was necessary, as Todd and Missy came by the hospital often. During the weekdays, Missy filled every request Kevin had for his favorite sandwiches, salsa, and yogurt. He was well cared for. On the weekends, Brooke, Regan, or I came and stayed with him. Weeks passed, and I learned more about patience than I ever wanted to. I read, *"Patience is not just the ability to wait, it's the courage to endure the waiting without losing hope."*

Waiting is hard.

Chapter 10

WORDS

Words Are Heavy

The roller coaster of information we received from the various parties at the U of M made the wait even more difficult. The case coordinator told Kevin to be prepared to wait up to a year for a new heart! That was devastating to hear considering we had convinced ourselves we could get a call at any moment. Dr. Roukoz was still entertaining the idea of an LVAD device for Kevin. This option involved an artificial heart pump device to keep the patient healthy while waiting for a heart. It is sometimes called the "bridge to transplant." That was not the course we had any interest in once we had wrapped our heads around the notion of a heart transplant. The weight of people's words on a sick person's psyche are heavy. We would dissect every conversation looking for a glimmer of hope.

I don't remember when Kevin and I consciously made this decision but we both really wanted to remain in unity on any decisions we would face. When an opinion by a doctor or any other medical professional would conflict, we decided Dr. Cogswell was the one we were going to trust. That decision became very important for our mental health. We both trusted her. She was straightforward with us and I sensed she really cared about Kevin. "From now on, if Cogswell says it, we will run with it."

No Mood for Small Talk

We celebrated our 31st Wedding Anniversary apart. Kevin was in the hospital waiting for a heart transplant and I was finishing up the last days of school. Later in the day I received a call from a nice lady from church who was carrying out her volunteer duty of calling people on their birthdays or anniversaries. I couldn't even fake being nice to this woman. It hit me wrong. I had no patience for her kind voice. I regret how short I was with her, but I just couldn't handle her sweetness. I had a similar response at the grocery store when the kind checker would try to strike up a conversation with me by asking, "Do you have any plans for the weekend?" I couldn't tolerate that kind of meaningless small talk. It would make me angry, and if I did try to sugarcoat it and answer, I always teared up. To this day, I am very sensitive to small talk with strangers because you just never know what someone is going through.

I also struggled with people's opinions about what I should be doing. Should I be in Minneapolis waiting this out in the hospital with Kevin? Bobbi called him every day and that was a huge blessing for him. My kids supported my decision to finish out the school year and be at home and their opinion mattered most to me. Our case coordinator told me to do all I could to keep myself mentally and physically healthy pre-transplant because after the transplant I would need to be ready to carry a heavy load.

Life-or-Death Decisions

It was a Thursday, and I was on the phone with Kevin. Dr. Cogswell came into his room and asked to speak to both of us. Kevin put me on speaker. She started with, "I don't know if you guys would even consider this, but I have a colleague at Baylor in Dallas, TX. I could make a phone call for you to see if they would consider taking you." The wait time in Dallas could be shorter mostly because of their larger population. "There is no guarantee they would consider the transfer and again we cannot predict the wait time," she added.

Immediately Kevin and I agreed that we were interested. Kevin was getting weaker every day he spent in the hospital. Cogswell never said it but I sensed she didn't think Kevin would make it if he had to wait a year. Remember: if Cogswell spoke, we ran with it.

This conversation got our hopes up. But once again, we would have to wait. First, we waited for Dr. Cogswell to get the approval from Baylor to accept him. She eventually got it. But then our medical insurance provider said they would not pay for the med plane to Dallas. Dr. Cogswell told us to be patient and let her continue to work on insurance, saying, *"I just need to get to one decision maker at your insurance company with some reasoning abilities."* In the meantime, we started pooling together resources, just in case. Med planes aren't cheap.

As time ticked by, it caused a roller coaster of emotions for Kevin and our family. The situation was taking its toll on Kevin's mental health. He needed a breakthrough, and he needed it fast.

Chapter 11

ANSWERED PRAYERS

Journal Entry: June 2, 2018

The Lord is close to the brokenhearted. There is a depth to life that you can only experience through difficult stuff. Some days I can view this process as an adventure because of the great people we meet along the way and the encouragement we can offer to others. How long did I live my life where I was just living one mundane day after another, all the while gathering information without transformation? Information does not equal transformation.

Brooke and I made it through to the last day of school and headed to Minneapolis to stay indefinitely. The decision to go to Dallas was still pending. Regan joined us and we all attended my niece Katie's high school graduation party. A little normalcy was good.

In a previous hospital stay at the U of M, Kevin and I had met Bob and Betsy. Bob had had a heart transplant and we met him walking the halls on day 10 after his surgery. We were amazed at his progress. Betsy and I quickly became friends. We exchanged numbers and became support for one another. She was much further into the journey than I was, and I valued her expertise. They had two beautiful daughters and we had so much in common.

Betsy had rented an apartment near the hospital, and they were heading home at the time we were waiting on the decision regarding Dallas. She insisted we move into her apartment while we waited. We took her up on her generous offer; it was a beautiful place to settle in. Kevin was of course in the hospital, but the girls and I were within walking distance. The apartment was on the sixth floor and had a small deck with twinkling lights. In the evenings we could relax on the deck and enjoy the view of the city.

After the weekend, Regan had to go home to start her summer job. It was hard watching her say goodbye to her dad. We didn't have a decision about Dallas yet and she didn't know when she would see him next.

Regan: I said goodbye to my dad at the hospital right after my mom had a slight mishap breaking a pickle jar in his room. The pickle accident added tension to the already emotional situation. I felt confident my dad would be going to Dallas soon, but I didn't know what that meant for me. The hug with my dad was a long one. He cried. Would I see him again? What if he were to get worse? Is there a possibility I will never see him again? I drove the four hours home and cried the whole way.

Journal Entry: June 14, 2018
This has been a very hard week in Minneapolis. It's such an up-and-down emotional time not knowing when or if we will be

going to Dallas. I am praying that a heart comes for Kevin in Min-
neapolis. Kevin felt crappy yesterday and I hate those days. I want to
trust the timing of all this but it's so hard. I will continue to pray for
Cogswell, her family, and her team.

The U of M offered weekly support group meetings for transplant patients and families. We had attended a couple of times. On this particular Thursday Brooke and I attended the meeting but Kevin did not feel up to it. We endured the meeting listening to other stories of success and life after transplant. We were still in waiting mode and also had the Dallas thing weighing on our minds. Brooke and I stayed quiet in the meeting and our mood was somber.

We left the support group meeting and made our way back to Kevin's room. While I was passing the nurse's station, Dr. Cogswell was behind the desk and on the phone. She began waving her arms at me to come over. She was on the phone with our insurance company and had secured approval for coverage of the med plane to Dallas! She ended the call with, "Thank you, I will go inform the patient." She immediately instructed the nurses to get the plane ordered and with a big smile said to me, "Let's go give Kevin the good news!"

A Warm Welcome

The patient and one family member were allowed on the flight. We were scheduled to leave at 3:30 pm. Brooke and I ran back to the apartment and packed. We called Todd and Missy to let them know we were heading for Dallas. The flight crew came to Kevin's room and Brooke walked with us to the ambulance. This is the move we wanted, but saying goodbye again was heavy.

Brooke hugged us both and waved goodbye from the door of the hospital. The ongoing uncertainty remained.

Missy picked Brooke up from the hospital and she spent the night at their house. Todd booked a flight for Brooke to Dallas the next day. Missy made a wonderful dinner with fancy drinks for the three of them. What an amazing support system! When you pray, the right people show up.

Support from the flight crew was equally amazing. Kevin's nurse was Patrick. He and Kevin talked the whole way and shared their faith with one another. Patrick's wife was the granddaughter of a pastor and he assured Kevin, "I will make sure you get on their prayer chain."

We landed at Love Field in Dallas at 8:30pm. As we were landing, I remember looking over the city and thinking, *Who is going to have to die here for us to have a happy future?* The idea that another family would have to experience a death for us to have life was very difficult and left me feeling torn.

Kevin was loaded into the back of an ambulance, and I rode in the front seat with the driver. She didn't seem to know her way around Dallas and the nurse with Kevin in the back was continually giving her directions. It was quite comical, and the driver finally admitted to me, "Three months ago I was a stay-at-home mom and now today I'm driving an ambulance in Dallas! My kids think I'm pretty cool now!"

The greeting we received once we arrived at Kevin's room was nothing short of "Texas Nice." His room was huge and there was plenty of room for both him and me. The head nurse welcomed him with, "Kevin, we've been waiting for you. We heard all about you and we're glad you are finally here!"

I'll never forget how wonderful it felt to be welcomed like that.

Of course, there are always issues to deal with, and in this case it was paperwork. The company that runs the med plane service required paperwork. I signed papers in Minneapolis before we left. I signed the same paperwork in Dallas soon after we landed because they couldn't find the first set I signed. The next morning, I had a message from the same service asking me to sign the paperwork AGAIN. I got a nurse involved to let me print my email and we finally accomplished what they needed. Those details fall on the caregiver. Insurance, disability, HR departments, phone numbers—all this falls on the caregiver. My binder went with me everywhere. I've been an administrative assistant my whole life, yet still my organizational skills were put to the test.

When we first arrived on the Baylor campus I thought, *This is huge. How will I ever find my way around?* I had just become familiar with the U of M campus, and now I would need to learn a whole new layout. Everything was overwhelming.

Psalm 23 helped calm my soul.

The Lord Is My Shepherd

The Lord is my shepherd, I lack nothing.
He makes me lie down in green pastures,
he leads me beside quiet waters,
He refreshes my soul.
He guides me along the right paths
for his name's sake.
Even though I walk
through the darkest valley,
I will fear no evil,
for you are with me;

your rod and your staff,
they comfort me.
You prepare a table before me
in the presence of my enemies.
You anoint my head with oil;
my cup overflows.
Surely your goodness and love will follow me
all the days of my life,
and I will dwell in the house of the Lord
forever.

Psalm 23

Kevin being loaded
into the ambulance on
our way to Dallas.

Chapter 12

PREPARATIONS BEGIN

I spent the first night sleeping in Kevin's room. It was huge, and there was a decent-sized cot in the corner for me. The next morning, we had lots of visitors. The case coordinator came by to get her necessary requirements done and she recommended hotel accommodations for the long haul. We had our first introduction to Dr. Shelley Hall, the head of Cardiology, and she brought with her two surgeons. One of them would be doing Kevin's surgery. Our first impression of Dr. Hall was all we had been told it would be. She was very confident and in control. She also wore beautiful shoes so I liked her immediately. The surgeons both praised her highly and we could tell she was well respected. I had a strong feeling that these two female cardiologists, Dr. Rebecca Cogswell and Dr. Shelley Hall, would become my heroines.

Prior to arriving at Baylor, Kevin had spent 36 days hospitalized in Minneapolis. Those 36 days transferred with him to Dallas and, according to Dr. Hall, they would improve his chances of being high on the transplant list. For transplants, it is not a *first come, first served* basis. There are many factors involved in finding the right donor. The patient's sex, size, blood type, previous infections, and health are qualifying factors. The health of the recipient is also a factor.

On the first day in Dallas, Kevin underwent a Swan-Gantz procedure. Dr. Shelley Hall was the surgeon; it involved a thin tube inserted in the neck into the right side of the heart for the purpose of monitoring the heart's function and pressures. I watched the procedure and I'm glad they did it to Kevin and not me. He had a big tube sticking out of his neck and it looked uncomfortable. It was a necessary requirement for monitoring his heart and keeping him on the transplant list.

Kevin was again blessed with many wonderful nurses. On this day, his nurse was Trish. She usually worked on another floor of the hospital but was floating to Cardiac ICU. We enjoyed getting to know her and she was very interested in Kevin's story. She read in the patient notes that Kevin was potentially the #1 person on the waiting list, and she couldn't believe she was going to be the one to take care of "that guy." She jokingly told Kevin, *"If you get the call, I am outta here! Preparing patients for a transplant is out of my league!"*

Once things settled down and the necessary meet and greets were out of the way, I set out to find a place to stay for the next few weeks. Baylor has a wonderful after-transplant apartment arrangement with a nearby apartment complex. It is called the Twice Blessed House. I had been in communication with them before we left Minneapolis to get on their list, however we couldn't move in until after the transplant surgery. In the meantime, I took the coordinator's advice and made my way to an extended stay hotel across the street from the hospital.

When I walked out of the hospital doors and felt the warm Texas air and heard the birds chirping, I took a deep breath and thought, *"This isn't going to be so bad."*

The hotel was lovely. The man at the front desk gave me an incredible discount and accommodated my uncertainty in length of stay. While I was checking in, Brooke walked in—perfect timing! We found our room and began to settle in. We took an Uber to Walmart to get a few supplies. Our room had a small kitchenette, so we grabbed a few food items as well. The hotel had a rooftop pool. We spent Saturday getting an hour-and-a-half of sun, staying with Kevin, and walking around Baylor campus to get ourselves familiar with our new environment. Who knew how long we might be there? It wasn't home, but we were feeling a bit more settled with every passing hour.

Sunday was Father's Day. Exactly one year before, Kevin had suffered his first episode of V-tach. What a year it had been! Brooke and I were glad to be with Kevin, but Bobbi and Regan were in Sioux Falls taking care of our sick dog, Bella, who had bladder issues. They were anxiously awaiting news from us, but we didn't have any. All we wanted was a normal holiday together at home, but instead we were miles apart praying that Kevin would get a new heart. How much longer, Lord?

Chapter 13

THE WAIT IS OVER

Monday, June 18, 2018

The day went by without any news. But the night was one I will never forget. Brooke and I had gone back to our hotel and settled in to watch "The Bachelor." We were in conversation about the TV show when Kevin called. We had just left the hospital; what did he want now? Was he checking on us to make sure we made it back to the hotel safely?

I answered, "Hello?"

There was a long pause. "Um Lori, they have a heart for me."

"NO, REALLY?" was my reaction. It couldn't be.

Once I realized he was serious, I started running around the room, pumping my arms in the air, and yelling, "YES, YES, YES!"

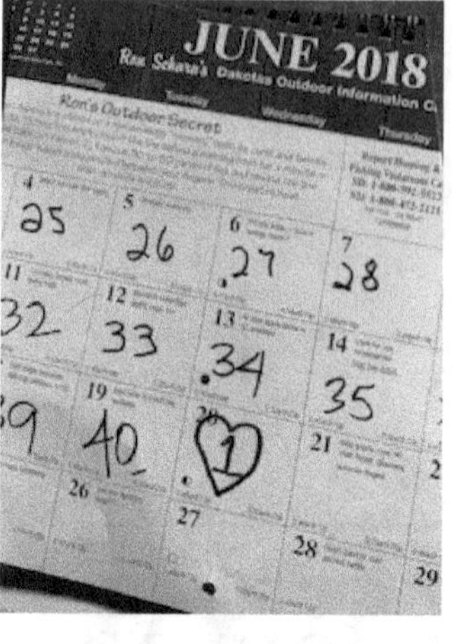

Our hospital calendar:
40 days of waiting

We had barely settled in to begin our wait in Dallas and now we had a heart already! We had been in Dallas for four days. He would receive his heart on day 40.

Forty days of waiting.

The transplant team had tried to call Kevin to inform him of the available heart, but he saw the call and suspected it was spam. He ignored the call. A doctor peeked his head in Kevin's room and asked him, "Kevin, are you answering your phone? We have a heart for you."

Brooke and I quickly made our way back to the hospital. Kevin was on the phone with his brother and had already talked to his sister. We needed to get Bobbi and Regan to Dallas asap. Brooke called Bobbi and I called Regan. Bobbi had just landed in Denver after her weekend in Sioux Falls.

Todd and Missy jumped in and put together flights for the girls as fast as they could. It was an adrenaline rush like I had never experienced. This is what we had been waiting for! I was somewhat afraid to be excited about this. What if the surgery doesn't work? What if we find out the heart is not viable? (It's called a "dry run" and it does happen).

Regan: It was a Monday night and my mom called me. She never calls me. I always call her. She calmly said, "They have a heart for Dad. We need to get you to Dallas. Call your uncle Todd and he will make arrangements for you." We said we loved each other and hung up. I was in my bedroom, and I fell to the floor. I was so grateful for this answer to our prayers. I didn't feel guilty for my times of doubt because now I was filled with gratitude. After a quick conversation with my uncle Todd, I had a flight booked for early the next morning. I was going to Dallas and my dad was getting a new heart!!

Bobbi: Brooke called me and said, "You won't believe this, but they already have a heart for Dad!" I answered the call while in the car on the way home from the airport. I had just returned home from a trip to Sioux Falls, so I asked Sam to turn the car around and get me back to the airport. I tried to get a flight out that night, but it didn't work. I booked a flight for the next morning and proceeded home where I spent a short, sleepless night running scenarios through my head. I wanted to be there before Dad went into surgery. I talked to him on the phone, but I wanted to be there in person.

The surgery was scheduled for 6 AM. Once we had the girls' flights figured out, we settled down. Brooke curled up on the cot in Kevin's hospital room and I laid in the hospital bed with Kevin. He had headphones on most of the night listening to Christian music. Neither of us slept and we each kept our thoughts to ourselves. I didn't allow myself to think the scary thoughts. God had blown open the doors to bring us this far; he would see us through. A few times Kevin removed one of his earphones and said, *"Here, listen to this. It's really good."*

Finally, six o'clock came. Kevin had talked to Bobbi and Regan on the phone. They were both boarding planes. He talked to Todd and Sheila too. We were ready. I expected more of a production in the hospital room to get him ready but instead two nurses came in and said, *"Hi, Kevin. Are ya ready?"*

I had been listening to "Overcomer" by Mandisa and wanted to share it with Kevin right before they took him away. The nurses gave us time to say goodbye and I played the song for

Kevin. Brooke and I were emotional and once the song was over, Kevin said, *"That's nice, but that's not really my kind of music."*

Not exactly the response I expected, but oh well.

Kevin's memory of his stroll into surgery was looking at the overhead fluorescent lights and thinking, *"Well, I will either find out what a new heart feels like, or I am about to meet Jesus. I'm at peace with either."* He said he was neither afraid nor anxious, but felt a peace that was supernatural and could only come from God. It came with a confidence that everything would be okay. Less than three years later, on April 16, 2021, our dear friend, Mark Steinborn, would say those words and experience that same peace. We look forward to seeing him again in Heaven someday.

Brooke and I went back to the hotel to grab some breakfast and prepare for the other two sisters to arrive. Our kind hotel manager upgraded us to a huge room right before Bobbi and Regan got there. It was so perfect for all of us to stay in. So many people extended us kindness during our time in Dallas that I can't even remember them all. Several nights earlier, for example, Brooke and I went to the rooftop to enjoy the city skyline. A large family was sitting around the pool. They had flown in from all over to attend a funeral. We shared our story with them, and they shared theirs with us. We had an amazing time with this family, and I know they, too, prayed for Kevin. Kindness and prayers were everywhere.

Our friend, Randy Hanzen, texted me when he heard the news, "Of course . . . only Texas would have a heart big enough for Kevin Sheldon" I smiled. So true.

Chapter 14

TRANSPLANT SURGERY

Bobbi and Regan arrived at the hospital. The girls and I were together again; I was so thankful. A surgical nurse called me every two hours to give me updates. She had a lovely, sweet voice. Each time my phone rang, I steeled myself for bad news. It never came. After five-and-a-half hours the surgery was done.

At 2:00 PM we waited in a congested waiting room with lots of other families. Kevin's surgeon, Dr. Meyer, met us and outlined a positive report regarding the surgery. We learned the donor was a young male from the local area and it was not a high-risk heart. Our compassion and curiosity about the donor did not come until later. At this point we were just simply grateful. The doctor advised us that we would be contacted by a nurse when Kevin would be ready for visitors.

After several hours the four of us made our way to Kevin's ICU room. We were not at all prepared for how he would look. It silenced us all. His color was yellow, and he was on a ventilator.

My dad had died of lung cancer while on a ventilator, so this was very hard for us to see. I didn't like this.

The first night was rough. The girls and I split into teams and took turns staying with him. There was not much for us to do as his care team was constantly vigilant in watching his numbers and accessing the numerous machines attached to him. Regan and I took the first shift. Bobbi and Brooke took over in the morning.

Brooke: Bobbi and I went back to the hotel room and set the alarm for our shift in the morning. We sat next to each other on the edge of the bed and tried to comfort each other considering what we had just experienced. Dad looked bad. Really bad. Bobbi carefully asked, "Do you think he's going to make it?" We were both scared. What if we made it this far and now he dies?

The next morning, Kevin attempted to write a note. From what Bobbi and Brooke could tell he was asking for his "wife." Of course, he thought I was off shopping or something, never mind the fact that I had been there all night long. (Sarcasm was still my "go to" way of coping with stress.) After a few hours of sleep, the girls asked me to come back because Dad was asking for me and he was unsettled.

As it turned out, he was actually asking for apple juice but that was not possible with the breathing tube. I knew he was most concerned about the surgery: Had it gone well? I got down really close to his ear and said, "You got a new heart; it's a good one. You're going to be just fine." That is what he wanted to hear. He calmed down.

However, his post-transplant doctor reprimanded me. *"Not to scold you, but it would be best if you and your daughters didn't try to communicate with him right now,"* said Dr. Capehart. *"We need all his energy to be focused on healing.*" The doctor had Kevin's best interest in mind, but Kevin needed those words from me, and he heard my voice through the fog. He later told me that hearing my voice was his first memory after coming out of the surgery.

Not an Easy Recovery

The next few days were up and down. Kevin was removed from the ventilator but had chest tubes and a catheter. He was having episodes of nausea and constipation and he slept a lot. His kidney function was a concern for a while but eventually the tubes were removed. He would get up to sit in the chair but would shake like he was freezing. His blood pressure was too high. They made him walk a little and continued to constantly fine tune his medications.

Three days after the transplant, the surgeon, Dr. Meyer, stopped by to see Kevin. He was very pleased with Kevin's progress. This made the girls and me feel much better. We began taking turns hanging with Kevin so that we could go outside, explore the Baylor campus, and tour the local area. I even met up with my friend, Natalie, who was traveling through Dallas. It was fun to catch up and it gave me a sense of normalcy. Lord knows I needed it.

Five days post-transplant, Kevin was moved out of ICU and into a regular room. His body was retaining an estimated 25 pounds of fluid, so his legs and arms were huge and seeping fluid constantly. The stretched skin caused bruising and sores. He was supposed to walk three times a day with a walker around the floor, but it took a lot of prodding to get him to do that. Needless to say, he wasn't out of the woods yet.

Life Goes on

I knew the time with my girls would eventually end. I wanted normalcy back in their lives, but I was not looking forward to helping Kevin recover in Dallas alone. The time Bobbi, Brooke, Regan, and I spent together sharing a hotel room like a slumber party was very special. There were times I couldn't help but think about how we had wanted a boy every time I had been pregnant. And now, it was so clear why God had given us girls. He knew the day was coming when I would need all three of them by my side.

Brooke was the first to return home. She was in the middle of her coursework for her master's degree and had to attend class in person. She was not happy to be leaving so soon but we made plans for her to come back later in the summer. A few days later, Bobbi returned to Denver. Regan was around to attend the required education for caregivers with me. But then, 10 days post-transplant, she too flew home and became an attending nurse to our very sick dog. Poor Bella was being tossed around between friends and family and was not handling it well. She eventually underwent surgery to remove some nasty bladder stones.

So there I was, alone with my husband, his new heart, and now two binders: the original one and a new one I had received at the caregivers training. I wrote in my journal:

There have been so many things I thought I would never do. So many things I thought I couldn't do and yet I do them. God has equipped me for each step. I can do all things through Christ, who strengthens me. Philippians 4:13

Despite everything that was happening and missing my girls, I was feeling good and handling things quite well. I even started calling Kevin "Tin Man" because of his new heart. He wasn't in a state to appreciate my humor since he was not feeling well. In fact, he was rather grumpy. I'll be honest: in 31 years of marriage, it wasn't the first time our moods hadn't matched up. But surgery was over and the future was looking much brighter, so I just rolled with it. It would work itself out.

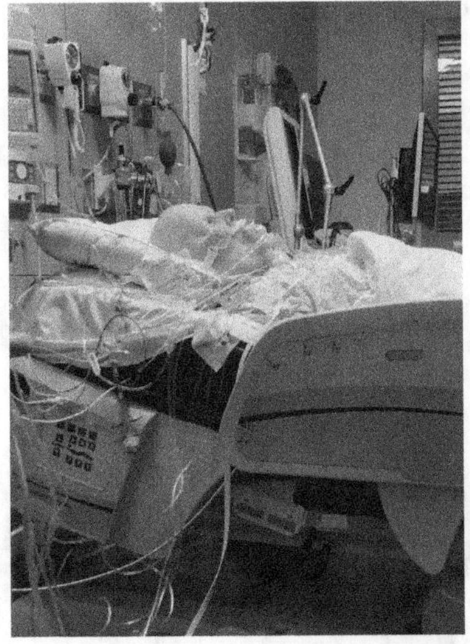

Our first view of
Kevin after surgery.

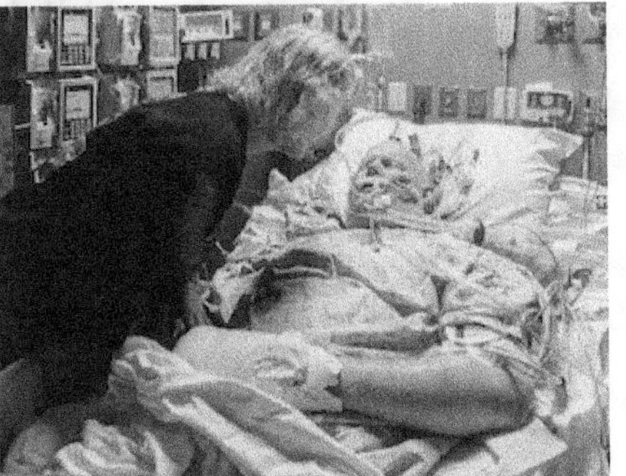

I'm telling Kevin,
"You've got a good heart.
You're going to be fine."

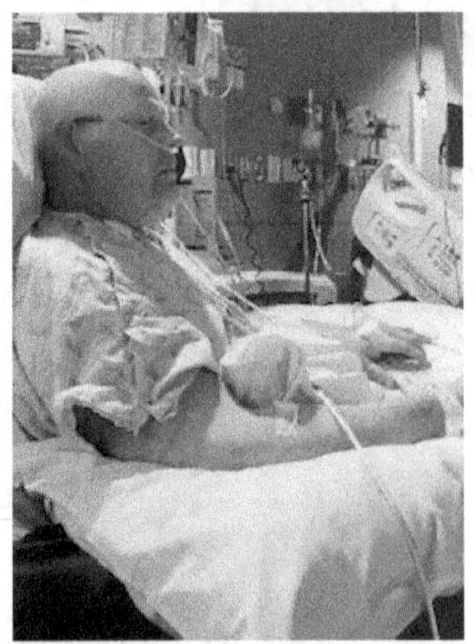

Recovery going well; Kevin to
be discharged the next day.

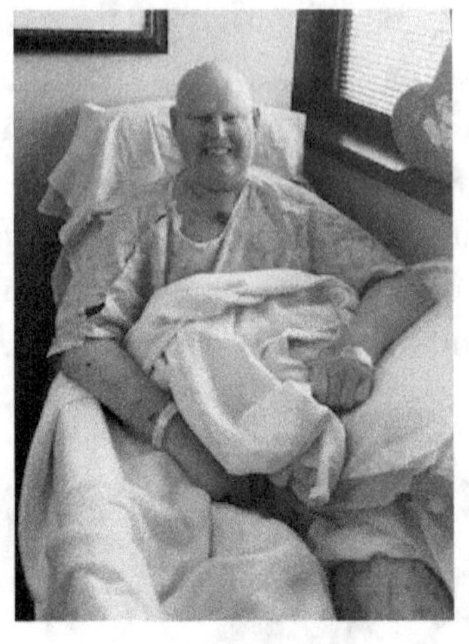

Sitting up in a chair two
days after surgery.

Chapter 15

DISCHARGED

After 18 days in the hospital, Kevin got news that he was going to be discharged. It was a Tuesday and I was lying by the pool at the hotel getting my hour-and-a-half of Vitamin D for the day. Kevin called and said, "I'm being let out today!" This was good news, but a lot of details needed to be taken care of. I packed up my things, checked out of my room, and left my belongings in a storage room at the hotel.

If you've ever been through a hospital discharge you know it is a long process. This was no exception! I made my way to Kevin's room and started the wait. The good news was that we had an apartment waiting for us at the Twice Blessed House two blocks away. The bad news was that I didn't have a car. I asked several nurses for advice on how to get him from the hospital to the apartment. One of them suggested a shuttle, another offered a taxi. We decided a taxi would work best.

The hospital pharmacist met with us to review Kevin's new medication schedule. It was intense. We carefully paid attention and it concerned me that we could mess this up. He spent a lot of time informing us of the things to watch out for, when to call the clinic, and when to go to the emergency room. Once again, I was reminded that we didn't have a car here, and we might really need one.

The nurses made arrangements for a taxi to pick us up at the front door. A transport escort came by with a wheelchair and a cart. I had the instructions on where to pick up the keys to our apartment: It turned out to be in an entirely different building. Thankfully, the transport fella was helpful and got us there. Eventually we made it to the front door of the hospital where we were supposed to wait. By now it was 7:30 PM yet still 100 degrees outside. Kevin was in a wheelchair wearing a flannel shirt and sweatpants and felt cold. He could not wear shoes because his feet were still full of fluid. We waited an hour and still no taxi. The transport gentleman made several calls on our behalf, but still no taxi. I decided to call Uber.

The kind Uber driver helped us load our things into his vehicle and also made a stop at the hotel where my things were being held. We finally made it to the Twice Blessed House parking lot. The complex had a large gate around it with a code required for entry. I began looking through the manilla envelope we had just been given with our key to find instructions on how to get in. Nothing.

I spotted a young man in hospital scrubs leaving the entrance gate. I jumped out of the vehicle, ran up to him and asked how to get in. He showed me the fob on my new key ring and how it would open the gate. Once inside the complex, I asked the Uber driver to wait with Kevin so I could go find our apartment. I started running and looking for #203. Once again, I had to ask for help from another tenant leaving his apartment. He gave me directions and I found it. Finally!

I ran back to the car and started unloading our things and throwing them onto the grass. I was concerned I had inconvenienced the Uber driver enough by now and just wanted to get him on his merry way. I quickly got everything unloaded from the car and maneuvered Kevin over to a nearby step where he could wait for me. I made several trips running our stuff from the grass to our apartment. Once I had everything moved, I said to Kevin, "Ok, it's your turn, let's go!" He stood up and was immediately concerned. He said, "How far do we have to go?" I propped up this 240 pound man whose legs were not strong enough to carry him, and lied, "Not too far."

We made our way to the apartment in the heat walking very slowly. He would stop every few steps and continue to ask, "How much farther?" Finally, we made it and I opened the apartment door to feel the cold air conditioning hit us. It felt amazing! We were in! Home sweet home!

Kevin got comfortable in the recliner, and I got busy settling us in. We didn't have any food other than some protein shakes from the hospital and granola bars. It was a one-bedroom apartment with two twin beds. The beds were not made but the sheets and bedding were in the closet. The bedroom window faced a fire station. Do you know how busy a fire station is in the heart of Dallas? It was constant activity all night.

The first night was not restful. Between the constant flashing lights and sirens and Kevin getting up every two hours to pee, it was rough. As bad as it was, I still felt at home because Kevin and I were back together. It felt right. Even my role as caregiver felt right; I had a real patient who needed me to take care of him. I could do that. In fact, I couldn't wait to do that!

After months and months of waiting and not knowing what to do, I finally had something to do.

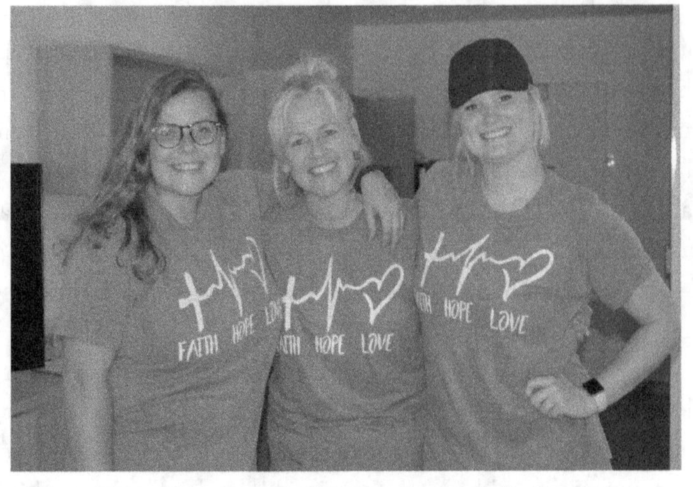

Regan, Brooke, and me in our matching shirts.

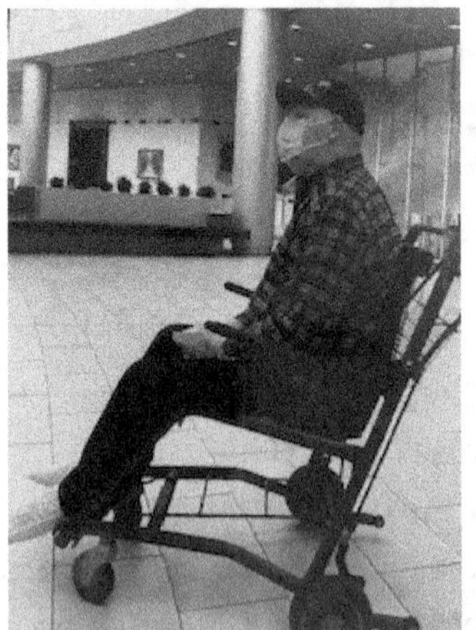

Kevin waiting in the hospital
lobby for the taxi that never came.

Chapter 16

WARRIORS

The next day was the 4th of July. I took an Uber to Target and filled the cart with groceries and supplies. I later learned that particular Target was in a bad neighborhood and not to go there again. While I was unloading my groceries from the Uber to my apartment, a neighbor across the hall came out, introduced himself, and offered to help me. His wife had had a heart transplant, and he was caring for her. I wasn't receptive to conversation because I was in survival mode. "Thank you, I'm fine," I replied. Some things about me just don't change: I can't be nice and be in survival mode at the same time. It's one or the other, but not both.

Part of the program in receiving a heart at Baylor is agreeing to stay in the area for three months for aftercare and rehab. We knew that and I didn't even let myself start counting days. Kevin had a long recovery journey ahead of him and being 11 hours from home was somewhat of a blessing because his only job was to heal and get strong. We had our entire schedule of clinic appointments laid out for us for the next three months.

Our first clinic appointment was two days after discharge. Of course, it was scheduled early in the morning because labs came first and needed to be drawn before Kevin ate food or took his meds. Keep in mind, I still did not have a vehicle, so I arranged for another Uber to pick us up. The problem was getting Kevin from the apartment to the parking lot. It was not far, but for Kevin it was. We put our arms on each other's shoulders and slowly made our way. I would sometimes think, *I wonder what I'm going to do if he collapses."* He never did.

I found a wheelchair for Kevin as soon as we got to the clinic. I had my new binder, a bag full of medication (the instructions said to bring it) and my coffee. It was all of 7:15 AM, yet it felt like we had already put in a full day's work! The waiting room was busy. We made it through registration and got checked in.

The lab person came and wheeled Kevin back to get started. I followed. Next to Kevin in the lab area was another man getting poked. He looked as bad as Kevin, who looked over at him and said, "What are you in here for?" The man replied, "I had a heart and a kidney transplant." Kevin thought to himself, "That must be why you look so bad." He asked the man, "How are you feeling?" The man replied, "Like crap."

The man's wife was waiting in the hall near me. I had noticed her in the waiting room because she was hard to ignore. She was more than six feet tall with gorgeous black hair piled on top of her head to make her even taller. She was wearing an orange sleeveless turtleneck tucked into her cute jeans. She had a large bag over her shoulder pulling the whole look together.

She tried to talk to me but I was in survival mode.

We proceeded on to the scheduled doctor's appointment and it was mostly uneventful. He was given a few changes to his medicine and some compression garments to help with his fluid retention, but that was all. I requested an Uber to take us home. During the wait, I parked Kevin and the wheelchair outside the pharmacy while I went inside to pick up the new medicine. When I came out, he was talking to the couple from the lab— you know, the heart and kidney guy with his six-foot-tall wife. They were exchanging phone numbers. My first thought was, "Ugh, what does she want?"

As chance would have it, they lived in the same apartment complex as us and they had a vehicle. She insisted we could call them at any time for any reason. Kevin put her number in his phone, and I thanked them for their offer but let them know, "I'm fine and we need to get to our Uber now." I simply did not know how to let myself accept help from others. I was in a survival mindset, in a strange city, and very determined to figure out the details on my own. Looking back, I realize my heart was in need of some healing, too.

The next few days were quiet. Kevin was sleeping a lot and I was starting to get bored. The Twice Blessed house had a catered dinner for us every Thursday night, so I took advantage of that. There was also a library for us to use along with a pool and workout room. Eventually I got so bored that I reached out to the six-foot-tall woman in the orange top. She had a name: Kelli Taylor.

Kelli and her husband Jimmy's home was in Benton, Arkansas. Jimmy's surgery at Baylor had been two weeks before Kevin. The Taylors became our lifeline and path back to a "normal" life. Kevin and Jimmy went to rehab together three times a week and Kelli and I walked on the track while the boys were working with physical therapy. We quickly developed a bond. Kelli is a nurturer at heart. She cooked for us, drove us to appointments, and entertained us, all while taking top notch care of Jimmy.

The process of getting Kevin's strength back required baby steps each day. He is a numbers guy who thrives on setting goals for himself. For a while, he even wore a Fitbit on one wrist and a Garmin watch on the other. His first walks were 100 steps a day within the apartment. He then moved outside and upped his daily goal to 300 steps a day: always about the numbers.

Kevin went to his first PT appointment in a wheelchair. By the second week of rehab, he was walking on his own and by the third week he was giving instructions to Jimmy about how to use the machines. Kevin's second home is the gym, and he has always enjoyed coaching others. Jimmy had been a roofer his whole life and Kevin described him as "butt-ugly strong."

The blessing of being able to work out alongside Jimmy gave them both the edge they needed to build strength and make a strong comeback.

The trainers at Baylor noticed the friendship between Kevin and Jimmy and the difference it was making in their recovery. The marketing department arranged for an interview with the two transplant patients—now friends—to tell their stories. The guys sat side by side while the cameras rolled, and the inter-viewer walked them through telling their story. Kelli and I stood by and watched. We were so proud of our warriors.

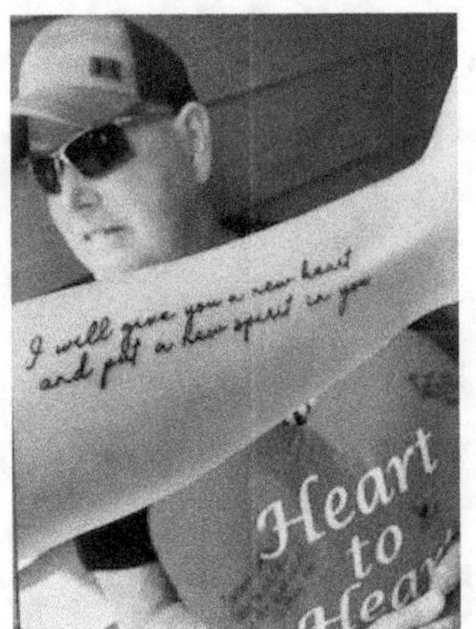

Our new friends: Jimmy
and Kelli Taylor

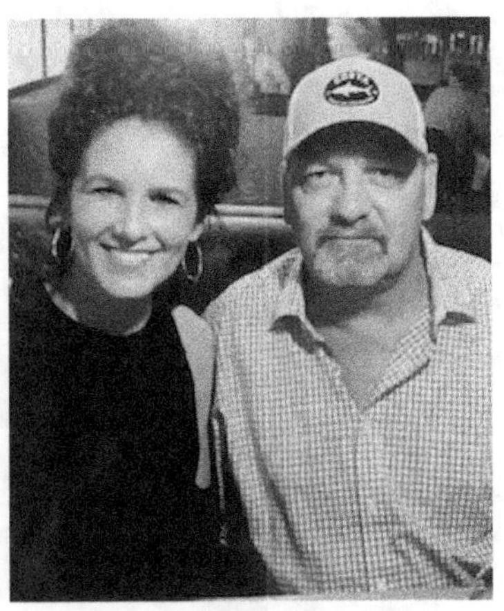

Daughter Brooke's
tattoo honoring our
promise from God.

Chapter 17

ALL THAT REALLY MATTERS

There were other transplant patients and family members at the Twice Blessed House. Every Thursday night we gathered in the commons area to socialize and enjoy a catered meal. Each week we heard updates from everyone and clapped and cheered when a milestone was achieved. It was very uplifting to be in a community where transplant life was "normal life," The man across the hall from us who was caring for his wife commented to me after several weeks, "Lori, I was worried about you the first day I met you. You looked tired and very stressed." He redeemed himself by adding, "It is great to see you smiling now and enjoying life."

I recognize now the loneliness I created for myself as a caregiver. I don't recommend my style of dealing with life's hard challenges. Everyone goes through hard times and if you haven't yet, you will. The whole concept of sharing organs between human beings is beyond my comprehension. I choose to believe it is part of our Creator's plan to cause us to depend on one another. In the end, our connection with one another is all that really matters. We were designed for relationships and when we try to battle alone, it is much harder. When we pray, people show up. It is how God answers our prayers.

We stayed in Dallas for three months post-transplant. As Kevin made slow and steady progress, we were eventually able to get out and do some "normal" things. My friend, Jacinta, lived in Dallas and made her home available to us anytime. She and her husband, Scot, had recently built their home with a desire to share it with family and friends. It was a beautiful home, and Kevin and I took advantage of their generosity. They entertained us when they were home and gave us a key when they were away. It was a wonderful and welcome getaway from our tiny apartment. Jacinta and Scot were truly God's hands and feet. .

Kevin was required to complete 18 sessions of physical therapy. In addition, we participated in a one-mile "heart walk" with 10,000 other heart patients and families through the streets of Dallas. As the end of three months approached, we knew we could start thinking about going home. We were so anxious to get back to South Dakota, but it meant saying goodbye to our friends, the Taylors. We had spent nearly every day with them for three months and our bond was deep.

Kevin's last scheduled appointment with the Baylor team was on a Tuesday. We anticipated being released after the appointment, but I was afraid to get my hopes up. He sailed through the appointment with flying colors. As per usual his nurse, Shane, called me later that day with Kevin's lab results. He gave me a few instructions for medication changes. I listened carefully and responded with, "OK, anything else?" He paused and said, "Have a safe trip!"

We were going home! I called Kelli and asked her for a ride to pick up our rental car. After scouring the city for any available rental car, we eventually scored a small Nissan pickup from Enterprise. We enjoyed one final dinner with the Taylors in Dallas, and the next morning we packed everything we had accumulated into the Nissan. It was raining, and we had an open box pickup. The Taylors helped us pack our things into garbage bags to keep them dry for the 11-hour road trip.

We made it through a tearful goodbye with the Taylors. Kelli Taylor gives the best hugs. I wanted to go home so badly but the goodbyes were brutal. We pulled out of the apartment parking lot in the rain and waved at Kelli and Jimmy standing on their deck. How could I be so sad and so happy at the same time?

The date was September 13, 2018. Kevin had not driven a vehicle for four and a half months, but he couldn't wait to take control of the wheel on this road trip home. The rain didn't last long and soon we were enjoying the open road through Oklahoma. Brooke and Regan were at home getting the house ready for us. Our friends, Lonnie, Diane, and Karen showed up to mow the lawn, spray-paint the lawn furniture, vacuum, wash windows, and shampoo the dogs.

We will forever be grateful for the gift Dallas gave us, but driving into our hometown of Sioux Falls was a beautiful sight. Everything about our homecoming was perfect.

Our daughters were waiting in the driveway. Our place looked lovely. My husband's heart was healthy, and mine was overflowing with joy, peace, and gratitude. It was all I had asked for, and more.

Philippians 4: 6–7: Do not be anxious about anything, but in every situation, by prayer and petition, with thanksgiving, present your requests to God. And the peace of God, which transcends all understanding will guard your hearts and minds in Christ Jesus.

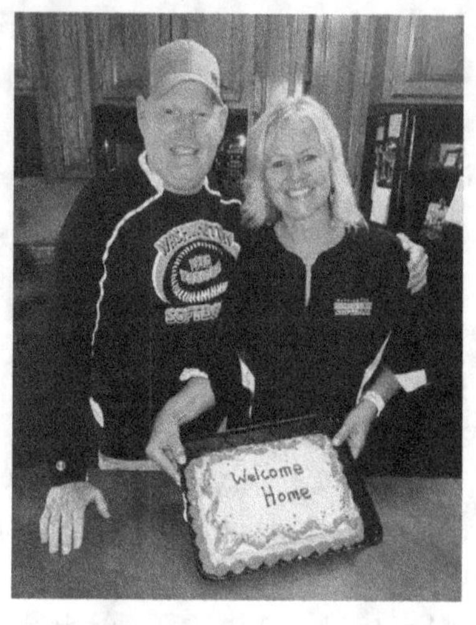

Our daughters had a cake made
to welcome us home.

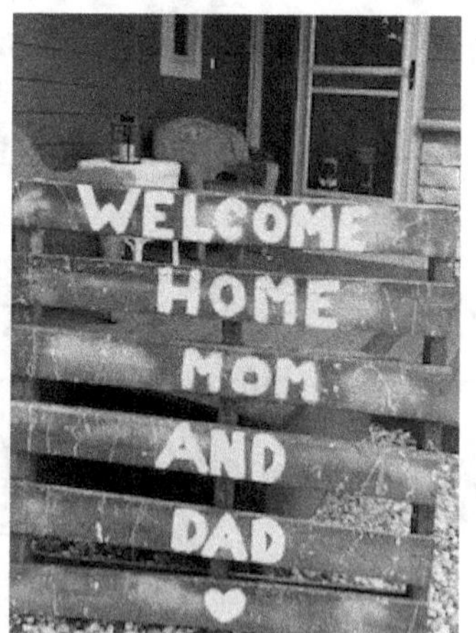

The sign that welcomed us home.
(Notice our puppies waiting at the door!)

EPILOGUE

Happy Fifth Heart Birthday!

In June of 2023 Kevin celebrated five years with his new heart. We've had an amazing five years. We love our story, and I am honored to be able to share it with you. Many people ask us if we have connected with the donor's family. We have not. The process involves reaching out through an independent organization to protect the party's anonymity. We sent letters after year one and year two and neither one has generated a response. We would love the opportunity to meet the family of our beloved donor. We will pray and wait. How would we ever express our gratitude?

Difficult times produce revelations that good times cannot. For Regan, our family experience drove her deep into her faith. The stamina and trust in the Lord this journey required of her awakened a desire to serve in ministry full time. She first dipped her toe in the water with a three-month mission trip to Zambia, Africa. Immediately upon returning home she realized she had to go back. God has provided a way for her to live full-time across the world from her mama and live out her heart's desire.

The direct connection between Kevin's heart journey and her life's work are stunningly obvious to us.

Last year, Bobbi married the love of her life, Sam. Kevin had the honor of walking her down the aisle. When I watched the beautiful sight of them walking down the staircase on her wedding day, for a split second I thought, "That could have been me walking with her; I'm so glad Kevin is here to do it." It was a proud moment for him, and Bobbi held on tight to her strong dad as she made her way to her future husband. Our dear friend, Lonnie Nichols, officiated at the wedding, and he gracefully weaved our family miracle into the service. It was a very special day for all of us.

Our middle daughter, Brooke, is a third grade teacher in Sioux Falls. We are not surprised she chose teaching as her life's work. Her "kids" are very important to her and she pours into them every day. But best of all, she too found and married the love of her life. Ryan is an answer to our prayers for Brooke. (Thank goodness for Bumble!) In August they exchanged wedding vows in front of family and friends. Kevin's father-of-the-bride speech reminded us of the many ways God has been by our side through life's difficulties. Two years ago, Ryan lost his dad rather suddenly after a short illness. We continue to pray for his family as they do their best to move on while honoring their missing pillar.

As for Kevin, he is back in his routine. He is working at a job he loves, fishing any chance he can, and back to his gym life. He enjoys working in the garden, taking an occasional bike ride, and finds joy and contentment in quiet, everyday living.

After watching my husband go through a heart transplant, I realize that tomorrow is never promised. I feel God putting it on my heart to encourage others who are in my shoes, riding shotgun as their loved one fights for his or her life. I am also aware that not all health journeys have a happy ending. I am sensitive to and very mindful of that harsh reality for many families, and I'm so sorry for your loss. I have lived with the uncertainty of a good outcome and because of that I am overwhelmed with gratitude.

Below are some of my lessons learned, bible verses that spoke to me, and a prayer of gratitude for the times when you don't know what to say. I hope they can be of much encouragement to you.

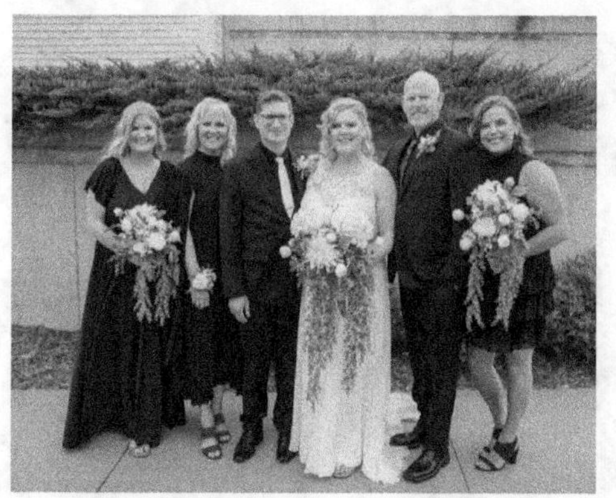

A proud father on Bobbi's wedding day.

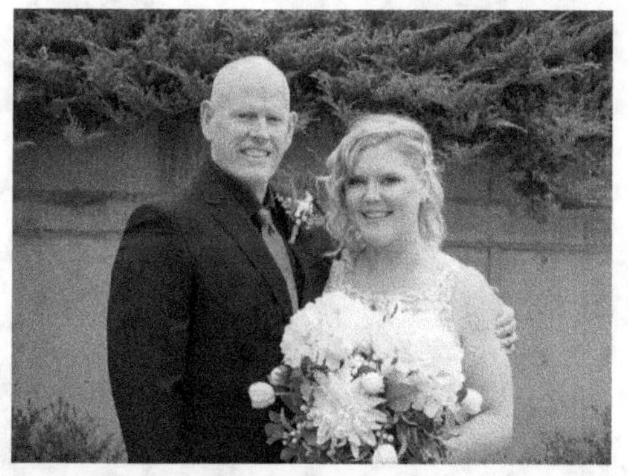

Bobbi and Sam's wedding day

Brooke and Ryan's wedding day

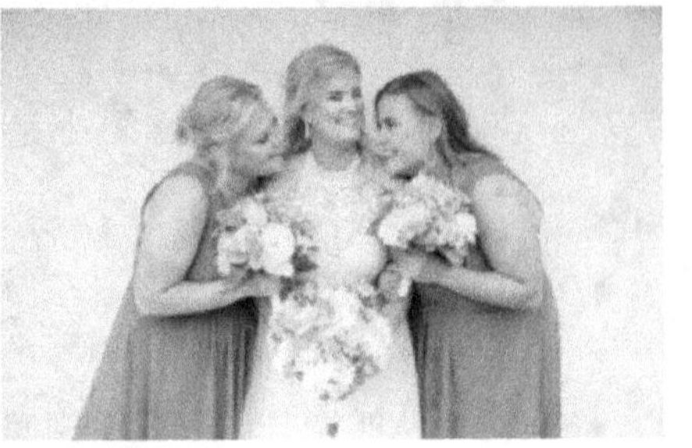

The Girls: Bobbi,
Brooke, and Regan

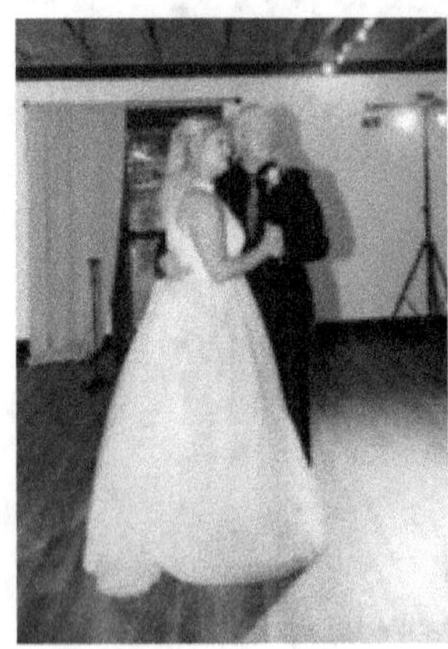

Kevin dancing with Brooke for
the Father-Daughter dance.

EPILOGUE

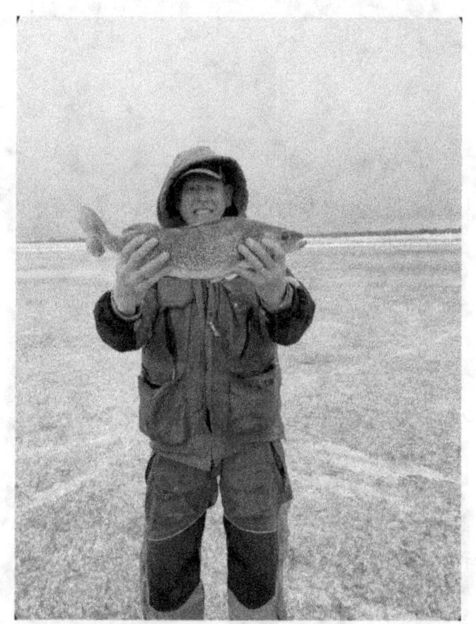

Dr. Rebecca Cogswell and Kevin

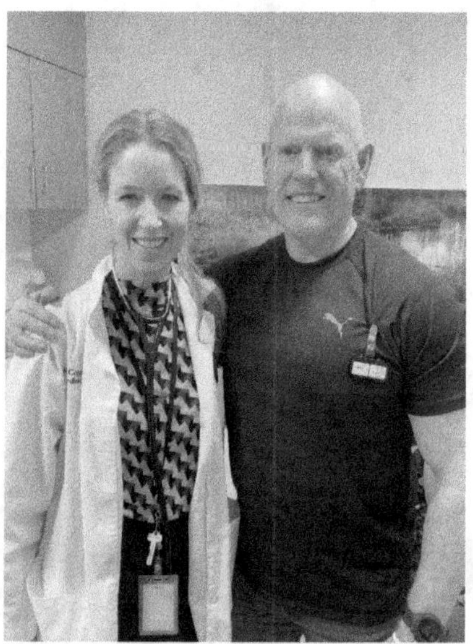

Kevin back to doing what
he loves . . . ice fishing.

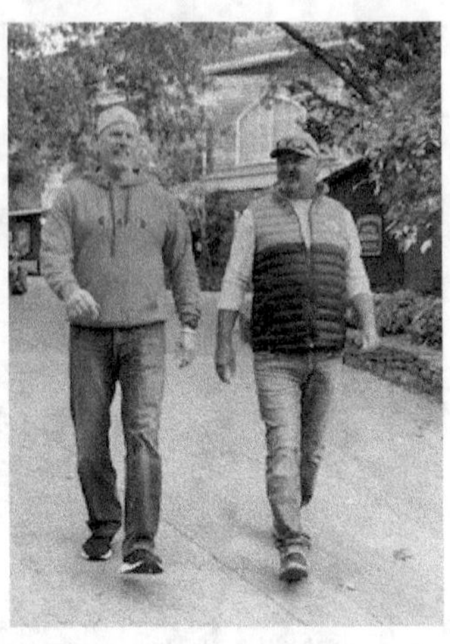

Kevin and Jimmy Taylor,
both living healthy lives
with new hearts.

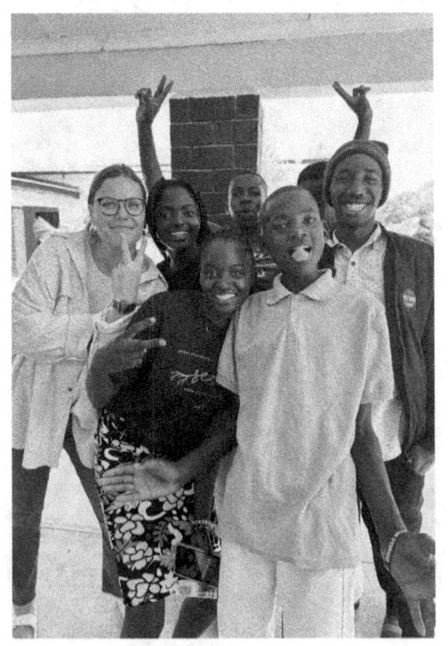

Regan living her best life in Zambia.

LESSONS LEARNED DURING TIMES OF UNCERTAINTY

- Pray. And pray some more. If you are too scared or tired to pray, keep it simple. The prayers of others will carry you.
- Don't be afraid to pray big. Pray and watch. God uses people to answer prayers.
- Stay in God's word daily by reading the bible or a daily devotional. I journaled alongside my daily reading. Reading and reflecting can renew your strength and bring peace.
- Be careful when researching Dr. Google. It can become a real obsession in an effort to find answers and to feel in control. Dr. Google can create fear—and fear is a liar.
- Accept the realities of your situation. Staying in denial does not help the person you love or the people trained and trying to help. The sooner you can accept the situation, the sooner you can get organized (aka: binder), and begin recruiting your support system.
- Come to an agreement on whose medical opinion you will listen to above all else. For us, it was Dr. Cogswell.
- If you take the time to notice, you will meet amazing new people along the way. Some are only for one day and others will be connected to you for a lifetime.

- Figure out whose personal opinions matter; for me, it was Kevin's and my girls'. Often I did not have the energy to fret over well-meaning opinions.
- It's hard to watch your kids worry. It's okay to let them know this is hard. What we are feeling and thinking is hard stuff. Acknowledge their fears.
- As a caregiver, step away and find normalcy sometimes. It's okay! I found time for walks, worked when I could, and even stayed home while Kevin was at the U of M waiting for a new heart. During these times, God still gave Kevin just who he needed.
- Be aware of your "buttons." Mine was small talk. Be careful not to lash out if someone pushes those buttons accidentally. They are social norms and life does go on around you. When life is hard, we are still asked to be patient and gracious with others and ourselves.
- Don't push people and their help away. This was the hardest part for me because I thought I could do it all by myself. But I couldn't, and God knew that. God used their resources, generosity, kindness, wisdom, and connections to provide us with everything we needed. You may be the answer to someone's prayer.
- Do something. It's hard to know exactly what to do when people you care about are struggling. JUST. DO. SOME-THING.

BIBLE VERSES DURING TIMES OF WAITING

- I will give you a new heart and put a new spirit in you; I will remove from you your heart of stone and give you a heart of flesh. Ezekiel 36:26
- Be still, and know that I am God. Psalm 46:10a
- Devote yourselves to prayer, being watchful and thankful. Colossians 4:2
- Do not be anxious about anything, but in everything by prayer and petition with thanksgiving, present your requests to God. And the peace of God, which transcends all understanding, will guard your hearts and your minds in Christ Jesus. Philippians 4:6–7
- When I am afraid, I will trust in you. Psalm 56:3
- Who of you by worrying can add a single hour to his life. Matthew 6:27
- My flesh and my heart may fail, but God is the strength of my heart and my portion forever. Psalm 73:26

GRATITUDE PRAYER

Father, today I am grateful for your presence and your peace. Go before me and make a way; stay beside me each day, and follow after me as I move forward. You know tomorrow, Lord, and I do not. Give me wisdom to see the opportunities you give me and the people I am here to serve. In Jesus' name, Amen.

HEART TRANSPLANTS

On December 3, 1967, Surgeon Christiaan Barnard performed the first human-to-human heart transplant operation in Cape Town, South Africa. The technique used by Dr. Barnard had been initially developed by a group of American researchers in the 1950s. The recipient, Louis Washkansky, received the transplanted heart from a 25-year-old woman. He survived the surgery and lived for 18 days. He died of double pneumonia.

According to the Annual Data Report of the US Organ Procurement and Transplantation Network (OPTN) and the Scientific Registry of Transplant Recipients (SRTR), more than 3400 heart transplants were performed in the United States in 2018. My husband was one of the fortunate recipients. Though we have not met the family who donated their loved one's heart to Kevin, we will be forever grateful to them. Their generous decision saved his life and blessed our family forever. If you would like to be considered as an organ donor, please share your wishes with your family.

TIMELINE

December 2013: Unusual rhythm detected by doctor and echo shows ejection fraction at 65%.

October 2014: First Afib incident. Angiogram with no stents. Ejection fraction at 30%.

2015: No hospital stays. A few incidents of feeling unwell.

April 2016: Incident at Chamberlain while fishing. CT scan performed. Found nothing.

June 2016: Hospital stay after doctor visit. EKG done and two stents implanted.

June 2017: Episodes of V-tach. Spent the weekend in the hospital.

TIMELINE

July 2017: More episodes of V-tach. Another hospital stay.

August 2017: First ablation with Dr. Pham (Sioux Falls).

September 2017: First day at my new job. Kevin is back in the hospital.

September 2017: Kevin is airlifted to U of M to meet Dr. Roukoz.

September 2017: Second ablation (U of M).

October 2017: Appointment with Dr. Pham determines another ablation is needed.

October 2017: Third ablation (U of M).

November 2017: Heart biopsy and Pet Scan to establish Sarcoidosis diagnosis.

December 2017: Kevin is retaining fluid and not feeling well. Kevin and I miss out on family Christmas.

January 2018: Trip to U of M. First meeting with Dr. Rebecca Cogswell.

February 2018: One quiet month.

March 2018:	Kevin wakes up sick. Another trip to the ER. Airlifted to the U of M.
March 2018:	Fourth ablation (U of M).
March 2018:	Evaluation for heart transplant.
April 2018:	Kevin is listed for heart transplant.
May 2018:	Kevin is admitted to U of M to wait for a heart donor.
June 14, 2018:	Kevin and Lori are airlifted to Baylor in Dallas, TX.
June 19, 2018:	6:00 AM heart transplant surgery.
July 3, 2018:	Kevin is released from the hospital.
September 14, 2018:	Kevin and Lori arrive home in Sioux Falls, SD.

ACKNOWLEDGMENTS

To my husband Kevin: You provided me with the material for my first book. No more material, please.

To my daughters: You redeemed all my worst parenting mistakes and turned them into three beautiful gifts to the world. Your encouragement means everything to me.

To Todd: I will need your gift of wisdom and calm for the rest of my life. Keep running, please.

To Karen: You know me better than I know myself. In case you didn't know, your number is #1 in my "favorites."

To Marilyn—my big sister, who would have been my biggest cheerleader on this project.

To my nieces, Debbie, Patti, and Lisa: Thanks for always letting me be your "sister." You are my anchors.

To our dear friends, Lonnie and Diane: You make us better people by your example. Our best times have always been with you.

To the many doctors, nurses, and coordinators that saved my husband's life: Your life's work changed our family's future. Aside from your gifted profession, you are people we cherish.

To my publisher, Jeremy: somehow your words motivate me like no other.

To my editor, Liz: Thanks for making my mess into work I can be proud of. Your counseling skills are top notch.

To my coach, Les: you held my hand and moved my book from a dream to reality.

To the ARMY of people who carried us: My biggest fear is leaving someone out of my book. Please know that every prayer was important to us and every kind word and deed were greatly appreciated. Because of you, I was never alone. You were all answers to my prayers.

ABOUT THE AUTHOR

Lori Sheldon is a South Dakota native, a wife, a mother of three and technically an introvert. She has journaled her way through most of life's experiences, good or bad. Her devotion to putting pen to paper proved valuable when putting together *Change of Heart*. Lori's career in administrative assistant roles provided her with the right skillset for managing her husband's five-year health battle. Her purpose in writing this book is to help caregivers and family members persevere during a long medical crisis when the waiting can seem unbearable and the outcome is uncertain.

Email: lsheldon@sio.midco.net